"Diabetes may be chaos, but this book brings some order to the daily challenge~ common-sense approach. The suggestions don't hinge on a given therapy or d~ obsolete in five years—but revolve around essential guidelines that will allow a~ healthy, pursue every dream, and thrive."

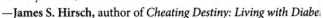

　　　　　　—**James S. Hirsch,** author of *Cheating Destiny: Living with Diabe~*

"At last, a book that talks about managing diabetes in real life, where stress from traffic jams, lack of exercise, and no-sleep nights happen. *Thriving with Diabetes* takes a refreshing 'life hack' approach to keeping blood sugar levels in range."

　　　　　　—**Amy Tenderich,** founder and editor of DiabetesMine.com

"*Thriving with Diabetes* is where science and heart meet. A handbook to tame your blood sugars, with advice from leading experts to heal your soul."

　　　　　　—**Riva Greenberg,** author of *50 Diabetes Myths That Can Ruin Your Life*

"In this must-read volume for anyone with diabetes, Dr. Paul Rosman and David Edelman take the mystery out of this most mysterious of diseases. The language is clear. The science is understandable. The messages are inspiring. With knowledge, support, and a bit of effort, you can indeed thrive with diabetes. This book will get you there."

　　　　　　—**Kelly L. Close,** founder of diaTribe.org

"*Thriving with Diabetes* is both the title of this book and the true goal of everyone living with diabetes. We work hard not for blood sugar readings, but to live our lives to the fullest. Dr. Rosman and Mr. Edelman offer many ideas for thriving, including two great strategies: focus on days where everything works well ('Use Your Best to Fix the Rest') and be willing to experiment ('Play With Your Diabetes'). Whether you have diabetes or care for someone who does, *Thriving with Diabetes* can help you achieve a life well-lived."

　　　　　　—**Jeff Hitchcock,** founder and president of Children with Diabetes

"As someone who has lived with type 1 diabetes for over 15 years, I know that things changed when I stopped thinking of sugar levels as random and unpredictable, and instead as a very logical physiological process in the human body. *Thriving with Diabetes* shows that diabetes management is not random, and with enough knowledge and patience, balancing blood sugar levels can become far less frustrating and far more predictable."

　　　　　　—**Ginger Vieira,** author of *Dealing with Diabetes Burnout*

"Living with diabetes is a 24/7 condition and *Thriving with Diabetes* integrates the most important things people with diabetes and their loved ones can do to live a long, health-filled life. This is a truly exceptional book written by authors who get it!"

　　　　　　—**Steven Edelman,** M.D., director of the Diabetes Care Clinic, VA San Diego Medical Center

"Empowering patients to make the best decision is essential for good patient management. *Thriving with Diabetes* provides the tools to make those decisions. Kudos to Dr. Rosman and David Edelman for reaching out in this way to individuals with diabetes and their families."

　　　　　　—**Jeffrey S. Freeman,** D.O., F.A.C.O.I., F.N.L.A.

With love to Barbara, who makes my world a better place every day, and our son Jefferson, who reminds me that the future is now. To Drs. David Goodman, Martin Sonenberg, and Elliot Weitzman, who made this book possible. To my students, residents, and fellows who challenge me to "keep it relevant." To my patients, who taught me that "using your best" makes sugars more predictable and dreams come true.
—Paul Rosman

To Elizabeth Zabell, who showed me the importance of approaching diabetes from a place of love. To my many friends living with diabetes, who work so hard to bring hope to others. And to Leah, who sprinkles every day with joy. —David Edelman

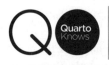

Quarto is the authority on a wide range of topics.

Quarto educates, entertains and enriches the lives of our readers—enthusiasts and lovers of hands-on living.

www.quartoknows.com

First published in the USA in 2015 by
Fair Winds Press, a member of
Quarto Publishing Group USA Inc.
100 Cummings Center
Suite 406-L
Beverly, MA 01915-6101
www.fairwindspress.com

19 18 17 16 15 1 2 3 4 5

ISBN: 978-1-59233-677-7

Digital edition published in 2015
eISBN: 978-1-62788-301-6

Library of Congress Cataloging-in-Publication Data available

Book design by *tabula rasa* graphic design
Printed and bound in the United States

"Keep Track of What Really Counts" and "Use Your Best to Fix the Rest" are, respectively, trade- and servicemarks belonging to Paul Rosman.

The information in this book is for educational purposes only. It is not intended to replace the advice of a physician or medical practitioner. Please see your health care provider before beginning any new health program.

THRIVING
WITH
DIABETES

Learn How to Take Charge of
Your Body to Balance Your Sugars
and Improve Your Lifelong Health

PAUL ROSMAN, D.O., F.A.C.P, F.A.C.E
and DAVID EDELMAN

FAIR WINDS

CONTENTS

Preface
Tune In to Your Self **06**

Introduction
A Personal Journey **08**

PART 1
BE CAPTAIN OF YOUR SHIP **12**

Chapter 1
Let Go of "Control" to Go with the Flow **13**

Chapter 2
The Thriving Action Plan **26**

Chapter 3
Take Charge with Knowledge **37**

PART 2
THE 4-STEP ACTION PLAN **65**

Chapter 4
Step 1: Lower the Highs **66**

Chapter 5
Step 2: Limit the Lows **83**

Chapter 6
Step 3: Use Your Best to Fix the Rest **98**

Chapter 7
Step 4: Play with Your Diabetes **119**

PART 3
THRIVE FOR LIFE..133

Chapter 8
Lead Your Health Care Team..134

Chapter 9
Change Your Habits...144

Chapter 10
Manage Your Emotions...152

Chapter 11
Banish Burnout and Diabetes Distress..166

Chapter 12
Build Your Support Network...174

Resources...185
    Appendix A: Letter to Your Health Care Provider..185
    Appendix B: Medications that Lower Blood Sugar...191
    Appendix C: Worksheets...192
Acknowledgments...197
About the Authors...201
References...202
Index...205

Preface

Tune In to Your Self

You can't tell that someone has diabetes by looking at him or her. Over the decades, I have confronted the enormous challenge of helping people succeed with this invisible condition.

Diabetes and its complications engulf people's lives, frequently impacts their families, and sometimes causes death. I have come to question whether we "providers" are doing everything possible to prevent these loses.

Early in my career, I worked on a team that created a computer program to predict blood sugars. But there are so many things that cause blood sugars to change that the computer ground to a halt. We were never able to predict blood sugars more than 90 minutes in advance. I felt like I had failed.

Over the years, however, I noticed that many people succeed in managing their diabetes. They don't just live with their diabetes; they thrive with it. I began to look for patterns. What led one to succeed and others to fail? Those who overcame the challenges had different diets, levels of physical activity, and personalities.

Yet, there were critical things that they all had in common. Each had found a personal approach that worked, even though the same approach might have been a total failure for someone else. They found ways to manage their diabetes more intuitively, to minimize its impact on their lives. When life got bumpy, they knew how to recover quickly. By making their diabetes more predictable, they were able to see into the future in a way that my computer program never could.

Step by step, I took what I knew about diabetes apart and put it back together again, uncovering the critical behaviors that separated those who were succeeding from those who were failing. Then I started teaching those behaviors to others.

In 2009, I met David Edelman, co-creator of the Diabetes Daily online community. He had, like me discovered that some members had made their diabetes predictable while others didn't know where to start. He invited me to collaborate on a solution. Over the course of a year, almost a thousand people participated in our Thriving with Diabetes online workshops.

We were deeply moved by the success of the participants and began another collaboration to bring you this book. The *Thriving with Diabetes* process has already helped thousands of people, and we believe it can help you, too. You can live a healthy and happy life—with you in the driver's seat, not your diabetes. Let's make it happen.

—Paul Rosman, D.O., F.A.C.P., F.A.C.E.

A Place for Connection

I met Elizabeth Zabell in 2005, two months after she had been diagnosed with type 1 diabetes. I vividly remember the way her shoulders relaxed when she discovered other young women writing about living with diabetes, working and starting families. She was not in this alone.

We started Diabetes Daily a few months later, believing that if we created a place for knowledge-sharing and connection, we could help others find solace, hope, and a way to thrive. Yet, as we participated in countless online conversations, we began to see that many people visiting the community did not know enough about how diabetes worked to be successful in managing it.

When I met Dr. Paul Rosman, I was feeling an urgent need to support our community members in developing the skills they needed to manage their diabetes and be happy. Dr. Rosman felt the same way, and we began to collaborate. This book is the result, a roadmap that anyone—regardless of their approach—can use to thrive with diabetes. I believe it captures the wisdom of those conversations on Diabetes Daily. Creating this roadmap is just the first step. We invite you to take the next one with us.

—David Edelman

Introduction

A Personal Journey

Thriving with Diabetes is not about sitting back and philosophizing. It is about action. Everyone living with diabetes knows it is an intimate condition. It cuts across every part of your life. It can feel like your choices are limited and all of your decisions second-guessed. On some days, it can be overwhelming.

We will show you how to reduce the burden of living with diabetes so that you can focus on living your life. You will discover ways of feeling better day-to-day, and also reduce your long-term risk of complications. Many of you will make your diabetes easier to manage, and if you have type 2 diabetes, possibly roll it back and stop taking medication altogether.

This book is for people with all types of diabetes, whether type 1, type 2, Maturity Onset Diabetes of the Young (MODY), Latent Autoimmune Diabetes of Adulthood (LADA), or another variant. It is also written for those who care for someone living with diabetes. The challenges vary among young and old, newly diagnosed and veterans—but that's okay. The *Thriving with Diabetes* process can help everyone with diabetes.

In this book, we assume that you have some basic knowledge of diabetes. If you were just diagnosed today, then you would benefit from first learning the basics of how to test your blood sugar, what foods contain carbohydrates, and other essential background information. You could get this information from one of the many excellent primers on diabetes, a class at a hospital, an appointment with a diabetes educator, or on the internet. If you have had diabetes for a few months or are already comfortable with the basics, this book can help you take charge of your blood sugars and your life.

Many of you have struggled with diabetes for years or perhaps even decades. Why should our approach work, when others have failed? Because in *Thriving with*

Diabetes, we recognize the critical role your body rhythms play in predicting and improving your blood sugars. We know it's not just about sugars, but successfully changing your habits.

Yet, while this knowledge has been validated by thirty years of medical, scientific, and behavior change research, much of it remains unused by health care providers and those who fund treatment. Consequently, most people with diabetes are unaware of the small but effective changes they can immediately implement to transform their lives.

Our premise is about self-reliance, rather than typical overdependence on doctors in a health care system that primarily pays to fix what's wrong, and hardly ever to find what's right. Using the tools and strategies we discuss, you'll be able to take charge of the highs and lows that can dominate your life, as Mel's story illustrates.

Even "Brittle" Diabetes Can be Conquered

Sometimes, people get so lost in their diabetes that it becomes completely unpredictable. This is called "brittle" diabetes. Blood sugars go on a dangerous roller coaster, careening from highs to lows and back again. This is what happened to Mel.

Mel was 34 years old and very sick when I met him. His life revolved around an unsatisfying diet, painful neuropathy, and kidney failure requiring hemodialysis three times a week. Over time, he had lost the ability to recognize his low-sugar reactions. He had a strong will to improve his diabetes management, but didn't know what to do.

One day, Mel arrived at the hospital unconscious after a low blood sugar. He was treated and sent home from the emergency room. A month later, he came back with another low sugar reaction that caused him to lose consciousness. This time, it took him three days to recover enough to be discharged.

Less than three weeks after that, Mel borrowed his father's car to run an errand. Thankfully, his father looked out the window of his house and saw Mel slumped over the steering wheel, the car still running. His father ran out to see what was wrong and found him having a seizure.

Emergency responders checked his sugars on the way to the hospital and found his sugar level was 22 mg/dL (1.2 mmol/L). (Anything under 70 mg/dL [3.9 mmol/L] is too low. If it goes too low for too long, it can lead to coma or death, sometimes, in just hours.)

After some investigation, we learned that Mel hadn't noticed when his blood-sugar levels crashed to 30 mg/dL (1.7 mmol/L) or below. These unrecognized lows were causing memory lapses. He would talk to you, discuss plans for the day, and not remember any of the conversation. When he did any physical activity, his blood sugars fell rapidly, before anyone could notice.

I knew Mel would die if we did not prevent these low sugars from happening. Fortunately, there was a new way to measure sugar levels using a sensor placed beneath the skin. Mel was one of the first people to use this new technology, called a continuous glucose meter (page 39). Mel's life was transformed when he could see how his blood sugars changed. Sensor readings appeared every five minutes on a laptop computer that he started carrying with him.

Mel was captivated by how his food choices and activities caused his blood sugars to rise and fall in predictable ways and learned how to respond before they went too far in either direction. He found that some activities made a big difference in his sugar levels, while others did not: watching television had no impact, but a morning of gardening would lower his sugars for several hours. Within weeks, he could predict when his sugars would drop and began to feel the onset of low sugars, improving his awareness.

Equipped with such knowledge, Mel had no more hospital admissions until he received a pancreas transplant that cured his diabetes, nearly two years later.

....

Thankfully, you probably won't need a continuous glucose monitor to figure out why your sugars are going up and down. In this book, we will show you how to get that information using just a handful of blood sugar checks.

POWER IS PERSONAL

The trick is for people with diabetes to figure out what causes their unwanted sugar changes and prevent them from happening. In Parts One (Be Captain of Your Ship) and Two (The 4-Step Action Plan), we'll lay out tools and strategies for tuning in and taking charge. *Thriving with Diabetes* is about more than managing your blood sugars. In Part Three (Thrive for Life), we'll look at ways to improve your habits, manage your emotions, and overcome diabetes burnout.

You'll notice that we don't make a lot of hard recommendations in this book. We don't advise you to eat 45 grams of carbohydrates per meal. We don't tell you to check your blood sugar six times per day. We don't decide how many minutes you should run, jump, and swim. If you'd like recommendations on these types of things, there are plenty of places to turn.

But deciding to work out a certain number of minutes per day or eat a certain number of carbohydrates doesn't get you very far. The fact is that people are able to manage their blood sugars across a wide range of diets and levels of physical activity. What separates those who succeed from those who fail is rarely their fitness goals.

More often, those who fail simply don't know why their blood sugars change or have the skills to influence those changes. Meanwhile, people who pay attention to their natural rhythms, and how their bodies process sugar, learn to manage diabetes in a predictable way.

Thriving with Diabetes can be a roadmap for your health care team, too. We have included a letter to your doctors and nurses about this process in Appendix A. They need to know what you are doing and why, so they can get on board and help you be safe.

Discuss the self-care themes of this book with your doctor or nurse before stopping, starting, or changing your diabetes treatment. "First, do no harm," we learn in medicine. We encourage you to adopt this spirit and err on the side of safety in everything you do in your diabetes management.

Now let's get started.

PART 1

BE CAPTAIN OF YOUR SHIP

"If I had eight hours to chop down a tree, I'd spend six sharpening my axe."

—Abraham Lincoln

Chapter 1

Let Go of "Control" to Go with the Flow

When listening to people talk about diabetes, you'll often hear discussions about "controlling" your blood sugars. But control is too strong a word for this. Even using today's technologies, keeping sugar levels perfectly stable all the time is impossible. In people with diabetes, the powerful systems in the body that manage sugars are functioning poorly, or not at all. The system controlling our sugar levels has over a hundred moving parts.[1] No one can control all of them.

Did you know that your sugar levels can double in twenty minutes[2] and fall by half in forty?[3] Checking your sugars every hour would not be enough to perfectly control that kind of change. And you are not going to check them that often. It is not practical or reasonable.

Using a continuous glucose meter, like Mel did, is not enough. It's what he did with this information, how he played with it until he could predict what would make the sugars fall to dangerous lows, and then prevent it from happening. How he got from A to B, from brittle diagnosis to manageable sugar trends, is the process we call *Thriving with Diabetes*.

The types of insulin and medications we take are better than they have ever been, but they can still take thirty minutes or more to start working. So even if you spot a trend in your blood sugars, it takes a little while to change direction.

When you react to sugars that are too high or too low, the event that caused the problem has already happened. Until you learn why the sugars changed in the first place, you cannot predict when it will happen again or prevent it from occurring. You will be living and working for your diabetes all day, every day. You need a better way.

Thriving with Diabetes means you can see the road ahead and nudge yourself left or right to stay in the center. You can focus on where you are going, not on driving the car.

We want you to look at your day—your trip to the gym, dinner with friends, or your lazy afternoon at the pool—and know how each of these moments impact your sugars and what you can do to keep them where you want them. You won't make one change and fix diabetes forever by putting the *Thriving with Diabetes* plan into action, but you'll accumulate little successes during each part of your day. These successes are unique for each person, yet they all lead to the same place—where you can live *with* diabetes and not *for* it.

FEEL THE RHYTHMS OF YOUR LIFE

Your sugars are heavily influenced by your body's recurring rhythms. During the day and night, factors like exercise, meals, stress, and sleep have a predictable impact on sugar levels.[4] When you tune into these rhythms, you can predict whether your sugars will rise or fall and often, by how much. Things fall into place when you can sustain your target sugar levels through the cycles of your days, under different kinds of stress, and during seasons of the year.

This is just the beginning. As you gain mastery over diabetes, you will feel more hopeful, gain confidence, and feel safer. *Thriving with Diabetes* is about taking care of your body to free up your energy to live your life.

GO AHEAD AND WRITE IN THE MARGINS!

To get the most from this book, it's important to use it as a tool for taking action. We recommend taking notes as you go. Grab a pencil and circle, star, or underline. It's your life. Take charge!

WHY AND HOW DO SUGARS CHANGE?

Life with diabetes is complex. A nightmare in the middle of the night can send blood sugars soaring. So can digesting food from a late dinner. Long-acting insulin from the morning before begins to fade. Every part of the day presents a unique set of challenges. We'll talk about how to meet these challenges in the chapters that follow. The important thing to know now is that blood sugars rise and fall all the time.

Take someone without diabetes and measure their blood sugar every few minutes. What do you see? Sugars rise and fall as their body processes food into sugar to be used as fuel (see figure 1.1).[5] And this is someone with a perfectly functioning pancreas! In someone with diabetes, the process is more extreme. The body can't naturally balance sugars, either because it's not using insulin very well (type 2 diabetes) or producing little to no insulin (type 1 diabetes).

Short-Term Impacts of High Blood Sugar

High blood sugars make you thirsty. As all that sugar builds up in your blood, your body tries to flush out as much as possible with frequent urination. This can wake you up frequently in the middle of the night. If you don't drink enough water to replenish lost fluids, you will become dehydrated. This can make you feel sleepy, lightheaded, and cause headaches.

High sugars also sap your strength. Your body has plenty of sugar, but it gets trapped in your bloodstream and can't make it into your muscle cells. Without fuel, your muscles can't function. They become weak. The lack of energy and interrupted

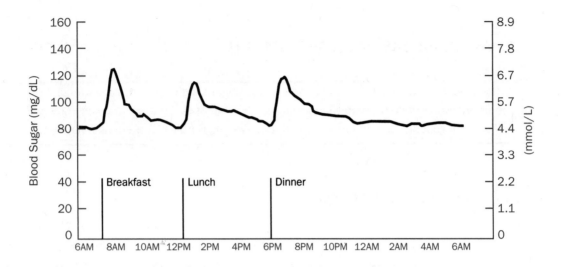

FIGURE 1.1 In people without diabetes, blood sugars change throughout the day, too. This is the average person without diabetes. Some will have blood sugars 20% higher or lower than this and still not have diabetes.[5]

sleep can leave you feeling exhausted and unable to think clearly. If your sugar has been consistently high for several weeks, you may not even notice that you don't feel very well. You may have gotten used to having less energy, feeling moody, being thirsty, and walking around with a full bladder all of the time.

Your body can become so used to high blood sugars that when you return to normal levels, you feel the symptoms of low blood sugars: shaky, confused, and generally unpleasant. Thankfully, these feelings go away within a few weeks.

Complications of Long-Term High Blood Sugars

Prolonged over decades, high blood sugars slowly eat away at your health. Diabetes is a progressive condition. Complications may impact your small blood vessels (microvascular) and large blood vessels (macrovascular). Often, complications are invisible until the damage has progressed significantly, with few ways to reverse them. This is why it's

LOVE YOUR BODY, FOR LIFE!

How you respond to diabetes emotionally greatly impacts your ability to manage it. It's not just about blood sugars, but how you take care of yourself and how you choose to live. There is a big difference between knowing the facts about diabetes and finding a way to manage it so you can live really well. Doctors and Certified Diabetes Educators (CDEs) can help with the facts, but they cannot determine what you are willing to do every day for the next three months, let alone the rest of your life.

important to take action now to minimize or avoid complications by finding an effective way to manage your blood sugars.

Not all people with diabetes will develop complications. While we don't know exactly why that is, there are powerful genetic factors at play. We also know that keeping blood sugars closer to the target range *over time* dramatically lowers your risk of short- and long-term complications, whether you have type 1 or type 2 diabetes.[6–11]

Unique Treatment

It can be frustrating if you have closely followed your treatment program and still experience complications. This is especially maddening if your prescribed treatment was destined to be ineffective. It's important to understand that just following a prescribed treatment isn't enough. The treatment must actually work well for you. If it doesn't work well for you, speak up!

Legacy of Health

It turns out that even a small period of better blood sugars can protect your health even decades later. We call this the "legacy of health." Multiple large clinical studies have shown us just how powerful that can be.[5, 10–12]

- During the 1980s and 1990s, the United Kingdom Prospective Diabetes Study (UKPDS) analyzed 60,000 patient years and showed that people can slow the progression of type 2 diabetes to reduce risk of major complications and death.[6]

- The Diabetes Control and Complication Trial (DCCT) studied 1,444 people with type 1 diabetes over nine years, ending in 1993. It looked at how "tight control"—aiming for blood sugars that are normal for people without diabetes—protected the eyes, kidneys, and nerves. Those who were prescribed more rigorous treatments did significantly better in all of these areas.[11]

- In 2013, a 30-year follow-up to the DCCT, called EDIC, had a surprising and encouraging finding.[8] After the original study, most of those who were intensively managing their diabetes had their sugars revert to their old, higher levels as they stopped aiming for the lower blood sugars. Yet, shockingly, this group still had fewer complications, including heart disease and death, thirty years after the study had ended. Similar outcomes were found in the UKPDS study in intensively treated patients with type 2 diabetes.[12]

The legacy of health is evident in the improving statistics on complications. A study from the U.S. Public Health Service showed the incidence of complications from diabetes

THE DANGER OF DIABETIC KETOACIDOSIS (DKA)

Short-term high blood sugars are rarely lethal. However, for people with type 1 diabetes and some with type 2 who are not producing enough insulin, long periods of high blood sugars can lead to diabetic ketoacidosis. The absence of insulin allows your blood to slowly become acidic. When combined with dehydration, this process accelerates into a poisonous cocktail that undermines the heart, impairs the brain, and can lead to death in days.

in America has declined during the past 20 years due to more intensive treatment of diabetes.[9] There are fewer amputations, less end-stage kidney disease, fewer cases of heart attacks and stroke, and fewer deaths from high blood sugars.

The Possibility of Reversal

There is more good news. Diabetes can be prevented in people who have a high risk of developing type 2 diabetes and reversed in some who already have a diagnosis. This was demonstrated during the Diabetes Prevention Program trial, in which lifestyle modification was more successful than medication in preventing diabetes in people with pre-diabetes.[13]

Regardless of your type of diabetes, daily choices make an enormous difference in your quality of life. Advances in our tools and knowledge have made it possible to thrive with a condition that for thousands of years was a lethal disease. Now, all types of diabetes are chronic, but manageable, conditions. And while genetics impacts your risk for complications, your blood sugars have a major influence. The little successes you will experience over the upcoming years will pay dividends for decades to come.

BE ALERT FOR EARLY SIGNS OF COMPLICATIONS

Complications may take years to develop in some types of cells, months in others. In some tissues, complications are reversible. In others, they are permanent. Let's take a moment to look at how the harder-to-reverse complications of diabetes begin, so you know what to watch out for.

As blood travels through your body, it branches off into smaller vessels and goes deeper into your organs. Eventually, these vessels become almost microscopic.

In people with diabetes, blood has higher-than-normal concentrations of sugar. The sugar can bind to proteins in the blood, causing them to get stuck. The smaller the blood vessels, the more damaging trapped proteins can be. When complications strike these smaller blood vessels, we call them *micro*vascular. Complications in larger blood vessels are called *macro*vascular.

Look for Micro Changes First

Complications often arise in areas with the smallest, most sensitive blood vessels. It can happen, for example, in your eyes when disrupted vessels bleed and obstruct vision. Left untreated, this complication can lead to scarring and permanent vision loss.

In the kidneys, damaged blood vessels reduce your body's ability to filter urine. The walls start breaking down, causing the kidney to leak protein and other substances into your blood. This can also cause scarring that increases blood pressure, which puts extra pressure on your heart and can lead to stroke.

Be Aware of Tingling and Pain

Tiny blood vessels in the nerves nourish cells that transmit messages from one part of our body to another. Sugar-bound proteins can damage the covering on the nerves. Initially, this can feel like tingling or pain. As it progresses, you can lose all feeling in

MICRO AND MACRO DIABETES COMPLICATIONS

Microvascular complications impact systems in the:
- eyes
- kidneys
- nervous system
- feet and hands

Macrovascular complications impact systems in the:
- heart
- brain
- extremities

those nerves. The inability to feel pain can lead to persistent injuries that don't heal or unnoticed infections that quickly spread. Missed infections—not diabetes itself—are one of the leading causes of diabetes-related amputations.

Macro Complications Due to Plaque

In the heart, brain, and large blood vessels, high concentrations of sugar change how your body processes fat. Fat plaque begins to line the vessel walls, weakening them. When these blood vessels are obstructed or break, it's called a stroke or heart attack. This type of damage can also lead to amputation.

Complicating Factors, Which Include:

1. Erratic blood sugar levels over a period of time
2. Genes that are individual to you
3. Lifestyle choices that impact your blood sugars or how your genes are expressed

Reaching and sustaining glucose targets prevents, and in some cases can reverse, complications. It is vital to take action now to prevent complications and, if you are already experiencing them, to put your best effort into achieving your blood sugar management goals.

KNOW YOUR TYPE OF DIABETES

Don't be fooled by stereotypes—both main types of diabetes (1 and 2) can occur at any weight or age.

Type 2

Type 2 diabetes is far more common than type 1 diabetes. It is diagnosed in 90 percent of people with diabetes, frequently among older people and those with excess weight. If you have been diagnosed but have never had diabetic ketoacidosis (DKA) from high blood sugars and are responding well to a treatment without insulin, then you likely have type 2 diabetes.

Treatments include eating fewer carbohydrates, increasing activity levels, and taking non-insulin medications, especially ones that contain metformin. Many people with type 2 diabetes also take insulin if their body cannot produce enough to manage their sugar levels. Going on insulin does not mean you have developed type 1 diabetes.

Pre-Diabetes or Gestational Diabetes

Type 2 diabetes is along a continuum as the body loses its ability over time to manage blood sugars. When this process begins, before it reaches the clinical definition of type 2 diabetes, we call it pre-diabetes. When the process starts during pregnancy, it is called gestational diabetes. Without action, pre-diabetes and gestational diabetes almost always lead to type 2.

If you have been diagnosed with one of these conditions, think of it as your chance to halt the progression into type 2 diabetes. Many people are only diagnosed with type 2 when they experience a complication such as nerve damage in their fingers, toes, or eyes. Early knowledge gives you a chance to slow, halt, or even reverse the effects of diabetes.

Type 1

If you have had an episode of DKA and take insulin, you likely have type 1 diabetes. This is more common in children and young adults.

If in doubt, ask your doctor to confirm the diagnosis with two tests. The first is a GAD antibodies test. When positive, it indicates that your body is creating antibodies to attack the cells that we know are damaged in people with type 1 diabetes.

The second is a C-Peptide test, which determines how much insulin your body is producing. The test requires a simple blood draw and should be done when your sugars are above 100 mg/dL (5.6 mmol/L). The C-Peptide test is not widely used, and should be done by a diabetes specialist or someone who is familiar with ordering the test and interpreting the results. It is not a perfect tool for diagnosis, as most people with type 1 diabetes continue to produce some insulin, especially in the first couple of years. If you have type 1 diabetes, the result will be below the normal range.

LADA

If you find yourself quickly moving from a pill to insulin injections, especially if you are in your 20s or 30s, you may have a variation of type 1 diabetes called LADA, for "latent autoimmune diabetes of adulthood." The treatment is the same as for type 1 diabetes.

POWER (OF INFORMATION) TO THE PEOPLE!

Over the past few decades, the ability for people to take charge of their diabetes has grown exponentially. "The blood glucose meter took power from the doctor and gave it to the patient," says Ellen Kirk-Macri, Corporate Nurse and Certified Diabetes Educator at London Drugs in Vancouver, Canada. Moreover, the internet gives people living with diabetes levels of knowledge and support that were inconceivable a generation ago.

This is the birth of the empowered patient. Led by individuals and medical professionals who are frustrated by our systems' failures, we are transitioning from a paternalistic, "do as you're told" approach toward one driven by the patient. This may be most true with diabetes, a self-managed condition where success is almost completely determined by the decisions patients make.

You may have experienced some of the ways the health care system is unable to support patients. Perhaps you've been to a doctor and been prescribed a treatment program that doesn't meet your needs. Then, to the surprise of no one, including the doctor, the program fails, but you are labeled "noncompliant," unwilling to follow the doctor's instructions. Is it any surprise that a treatment program that doesn't consider your needs, or provide you with the skills to succeed, would fail?

The disconnect is there from the beginning. You are diagnosed and see a doctor and then don't return for three months. Bear in mind that blood sugars change in minutes or hours. Learning to manage your diabetes successfully requires so much more than acquiring a few facts and taking medication.

If your blood sugars end up so high that you need to be hospitalized, the health care system will gladly pay tens of thousands of dollars to keep you alive. But it won't pay hundreds to take you from a place of constant mild discomfort to a place of thriving. And at the end of the day, that is exactly what you want to do: thrive.

Health care professionals speak of making patients the captain of the ship, but too often it's the doctor who plays captain. You must be the captain of your ship, and we'll tell you how in Part 3.

Understanding Points vs. Trends

As we work on making diabetes predictable, it's important to understand that a single number on its own has very little meaning. It's like looking at a single frame from a movie and thinking that you understand the story. Diabetes is not about managing individual blood sugars, but about managing how they rise and fall. This distinction is extremely important.

For example, your blood sugar is 100 mg/dL (5.6 mmol/L) and you are getting ready to drive. What do you do? If your blood sugar has been stable at 100 mg/dL (5.6 mmol/L) for the last hour, probably nothing. But what if it was 300 mg/dL (16.7 mmol/L) an hour ago, and you treated it with an extra insulin injection? You may be heading towards a severe low blood sugar—and possibly a car accident if you don't take action to treat the oncoming low by consuming carbohydrates.

Get into the Driver's Seat

Diabetes can be like learning to drive a car. The first time you get in, you're understandably anxious. You need to press the pedals, turn the wheel, and watch four directions at the same time. There are a hundred little details to pay attention to, both inside and outside of the car.

Though driving is scary at first, it can be exhilarating when you know how to handle the car. After a year in the driver's seat, you begin to internalize all these processes and start driving by intuition. You are focused on where you are headed, keeping a passive lookout for obstacles. You can safely listen to music, talk to friends, and enjoy cruising down the road.

One day, someone doesn't see you and tries to merge into your lane. After a quick glance in your rearview mirror, you tap the breaks and avoid the accident. Your heart pounds, but you feel really good about your ability to react.

Now, imagine if you never got comfortable driving. You were always hyper-vigilant, anxious about what lies around the next turn. You would never be able to enjoy a trip. You would never feel safe.

In driving and diabetes, there's tremendous power in going from a state of worry to one of confidence, from fear to mastery.

The key to this power is making diabetes predictable.

If your sugars have been a chaotic mess for a long time, then "predictable diabetes" may sound like an oxymoron. In these pages, we will help you carve your days into simpler, manageable periods and make them predictable, one at a time.

Chapter 2

The Thriving Action Plan

Many people who are succeeding in taming their diabetes are using the *Thriving with Diabetes* principles without realizing it. As you prepare to take action, it's important to ask simple questions and get simple answers you can trust and act on. We'll show you which questions to ask. But it's also important to find manageable ways to answer them. If you had to check your sugars 200 times to get an answer, would that work? We'll teach you how to solve problems with just a handful of sugar checks. You can often get answers in just a few days.

KEEP TRACK OF WHAT COUNTS

Are you recording every sugar? This could be a good thing or a waste of time. If you use the information to make positive changes, you are on the right track. If it isn't helpful to you or your doctor, then it's probably a waste of time, effort, blood, and money.

Harness Your Body's Rhythms

You may not be able to make your diabetes go away, but you can use your body's rhythms to your advantage. We'll make you more aware of your hormonal cycles and how to take advantage of them.

Err on the Side of Safety

When making a decision about treating your diabetes, especially if you are on insulin or sugar-lowering medication, there is an element of risk. You might have a low sugar, lose your ability to think clearly, and end up hurt or worse. One of the most important things you can do is err on the side of safety when making a decision. We'll talk about what that means throughout the book.

Feel Good about Your Decisions

Do you want to live your life for you or your diabetes? It's important to make decisions that work for you and that you feel good about. You can't ignore it, but you don't need to make diabetes the master of your life.

FOUR STEPS TO GREAT BLOOD SUGARS

Now that we've established some guiding principles, let's preview the steps you can follow to achieve lifelong success. We'll go into depth for each of these in subsequent chapters.

Step 1: Lower the Highs

No matter what type of diabetes you have, the first thing you need to do is reduce high blood sugars. As the body stops producing or using insulin properly, blood sugar levels start to rise. In Chapter 4, we look at many factors that raise and lower your blood sugar and put them to use strategically to treat and avoid high blood sugars.

Step 2: Limit the Lows

When you start to push your blood sugars down into the normal range, you become at risk for low blood sugars (also called hypoglycemia). These can be unpleasant, scary, and dangerous. Low blood sugars set off a chain reaction, releasing four hormones that work together to increase the levels of sugar in your blood. For several hours after a low sugar level, you are more likely to experience a high sugar. And when you correct that high sugar, you are more likely to over-correct and experience a low sugar. If you've ever felt like you're on a sugar roller coaster, this is likely the reason why. If you do not eliminate the lows, you will probably fail to reduce the highs.

In Chapter 5, we'll look how these high sugar rebounds act differently than a high sugar level after a bowl of ice cream or a piece of cake. Even if you are not on sugar-lowering medication, it is important to know how to spot and treat low blood sugars.

Step 3: Use Your Best to Fix the Rest

After you've limited the lows, it's time to harness your body's rhythms to minimize the ups and downs. In Chapter 6, we will examine the part of the day where you consistently feel good. Is it before lunch or right before bed? When do your sugars seem most stable? We will even help you find a place to start if you feel like your days are chaotic, which they frequently are with this intimate condition.

This approach is the opposite of that used by most doctors, who look at a list of sugar readings and pause at the highest or lowest to ask, "What happened here?" A more useful approach is understanding how you got the good ones and when they changed.

Step 4: Play with Your Diabetes

What to do when the unexpected happens? Or when the usual treatment no longer works? Chapter 7 will teach you to play with your diabetes and get an intuitive sense of when, why, and by how much your blood sugars change during a wide variety of situations. Life throws surprises at us: a party, a broken arm, interrupted sleep, chasing a young child. Learning to manage both the familiar and the unfamiliar are important life skills.

Once you get comfortable in new situations, you will get a good sense of how your sugars will react. Slowly, diabetes will go from an unpredictable mystery to something you have the power to influence. You will feel safe with your diabetes. You will gain confidence, feel good about your decisions, and feel better overall!

A DAY IN THE LIFE OF JOANNA

To be successful, it is extremely important to understand what causes blood sugars to rise and fall. Let's walk through a typical day for Joanna, a woman with type 2 diabetes. She takes fast-acting insulin at mealtimes to help handle her blood sugar spikes.

Morning Routine (figure 2.1)

Joanna wakes up, energetic and ready to embrace the day. After a quick shower and sugar check, she makes herself scrambled eggs on toast and takes an injection of insulin. She chooses her insulin dose based on her pre-meal blood sugar, how many carbohydrates she eats, and whether she is going to be physically active this morning. It's a quick calculation—she eats the same breakfast on most days.

Her body starts to digest her meal before the insulin kicks in. In ten minutes, her body starts converting the toast into sugar in her blood. Joanna's blood sugar rises from 140 mg/dL to 250 mg/dL (7.8 mmol/L to 13.9 mmol/L) over the next hour before slowly dropping back down towards 100 mg/dL (5.6 mmol/L).

FIGURE 2.1 Joanna wakes up, eats breakfast, and gets ready to go out for the day.

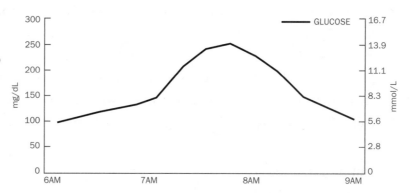

Surprise Encounter (figure 2.2)

An hour after breakfast, Joanna leaves to visit a friend. As she's driving through an intersection, a car runs the red light. She slams on the breaks, slowing enough to barely miss the car as she slides to the other side of the intersection. Before she even processes what happens, it's over.

Joanna's heart is thumping as her body floods itself with adrenaline. Within moments, her blood sugar is rising due to the "fight or flight" response. It quickly reaches 290 mg/dL (16.1 mmol/L). (She won't discover this until she checks her blood sugar before lunch in an hour, wondering how it got so high.)

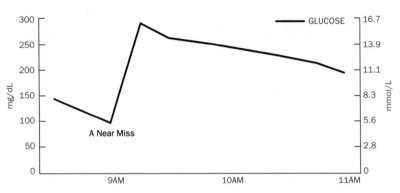

FIGURE 2.2 When Joanna almost gets in a car accident, her blood sugars quickly spike over 100 mg/dl (5.6 mmol/L).

Lunchtime Calculation (figure 2.3)

A little before 1:00 p.m., Joanna meets her girlfriends at a cafe for lunch. She checks her blood sugar and is surprised that it's over 200 mg/dL (11.1 mmol/L). But she takes two units of insulin to lower it and another three for her lunch and awaits the meal. Joanna laughs the next hour away with her friends. The food arrives twenty minutes after she injects, so her insulin is active and working as her food starts to digest. She enjoys her meal while her blood sugars slowly lower in the background.

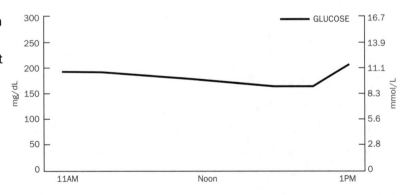

FIGURE 2.3 As Joanna sits down to meet her friends, the excitement causes her blood sugars to increase.

Afternoon Low (figure 2.4)

For the next hour, Joanna walks from store to store trying on clothes. It doesn't seem like exercise, but all that activity is making her muscles use insulin very effectively. Her blood sugars begin to drop faster than she anticipated. By 2:30, she's feeling shaky. She checks her blood sugar: 65 mg/dL (3.6 mmol/L) and dropping fast. She drinks a juice box from her purse and sits in the dressing room for ten minutes. She feels drained, though back to her normal self. She rejoins her friends, smiling but tired.

Joanna insists on stopping for a kiddie cup of ice cream. Checking her blood sugar, she's only risen to 80 mg/dL (4.4 mmol/L). She takes a little less insulin than she normally takes and enjoys every bite.

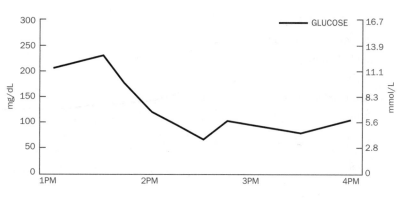

FIGURE 2.4 As Joanna walks around the mall, the physical activity lowers her blood sugar. She treats the low with juice and then later a little ice cream.

Dinner, Darling (figure 2.5)

Joanna says goodbye to her friends and heads home to make dinner. She is feeling tired from a busy day, mixed with the roller-coaster of highs and lows. She opens the door and smells dinner simmering on the stove. Discovering her boyfriend in the kitchen, she melts into a smile. She checks her blood sugar and sees that it's at 114 mg/dL (6.3 mmol/L). She's feeling good.

Dinner is chicken and vegetables sautéed in a light sauce. She knows that a plateful is reliably about 45 grams of carbs. She takes insulin, gives her boyfriend a kiss on the cheek, and sits down to eat.

FIGURE 2.5 After Joanna eats dinner, her blood sugars rise and then start to fall again as the insulin takes effect.

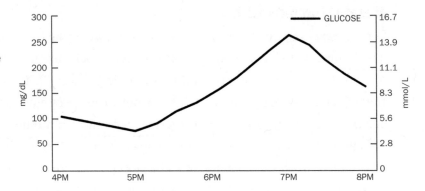

FIGURE 2.6 After dinner, Joanna's blood sugars slowly fall as her insulin works and she relaxes on the couch.

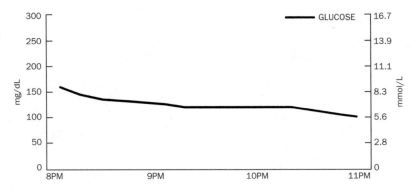

FIGURE 2.7 After Joanna falls asleep, her blood sugars slowly drop.

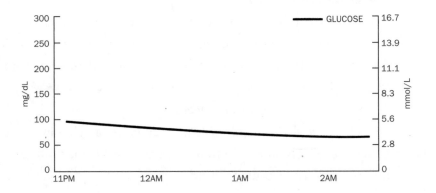

Good Night's Sleep (figures 2.6 and 2.7)

Joanna gets ready to sleep after an uneventful evening. She ate dinner and watched TV with her boyfriend and checked her blood sugar before brushing her teeth. (She's gotten in the habit of checking before brushing because it's annoying to eat sugar or drink juice to treat a low after she's just brushed.) She has a steady 120 mg/dL (6.7 mmol/L). About 15 minutes later, she drifts peacefully off to sleep.

As her body goes to sleep, Joanna's blood sugars begin to fall slowly. Her body no longer needs fuel for movement, so it stops releasing sugar into the bloodstream. Sleep is a vital daily period of restoration. Her metabolism changes in ways that will affect her blood sugars for the entire day that follows.

Internal Alarm Clock (figures 2.8 and 2.9)

About 90 minutes before Joanna's usual wake up time at 8 AM, her body signals for her liver to release sugar into the bloodstream. Her blood sugars rise from 100 mg/dL (5.6 mmol/L) to 140 mg/dL (7.8 mmol/L) in the hour before she wakes up. When her alarm goes off, she yawns, rises, and checks her blood sugar. Like millions of others, she is frustrated by the increase overnight. This normal rise in blood sugar levels is "The Dawn Phenomenon."

As you can see, throughout the day, Joanna's blood sugars are impacted by her body's rhythms, the foods that she eats, the stresses that she encounters, and her physical activities.

....

Find What Works: Mike's Story

Newly diagnosed with type 2 diabetes at age 73, Mike felt uneasy about his diabetes. He kept dwelling on his brother's recent diabetes-related kidney failure.

Mike spoke in broken English, with an accent that could have been Greek or Italian. After he came to America, he married, fathered five healthy children, and started his own granite business. Mike's business had grown, and now his two sons helped him run it. He was a self-made man and proud of it.

He followed his doctor's advice from the first visit. He went to a dietitian, attended diabetes classes, and checked his sugar twice a day. Mike found his levels were almost always above 200 mg/dL (11.1 mmol/L) when he checked them and didn't understand why that was happening. Dr. Keith wanted to help, but although Mike had been faithfully checking his sugars, he hadn't recorded them in his diary.

So, before the next office visit, Dr. Keith asked Mike to check his sugar level four times a day for three months. At the next visit, when Dr. Keith asked for the diary, Mike reached into his back pocket and with shaking hands took out a small piece of paper. On the paper, Dr. Keith found 336 separate sugar levels carefully listed.

Mike immediately pointed to the highest value, 358. "This was my granddaughter's birthday party. I had a piece of birthday cake. I was careful."

As Dr. Keith looked at Mike's list of sugar levels, he saw there were several days when the sugar level came down to 90 and 100 mg/dL (5 to 5.6 mmol/L). Dr. Keith pointed to these numbers and asked Mike, "What were you doing to get such great results here?"

"I don't know. I didn't write that down." Mike said.

"Isn't that what we are looking for?" Dr. Keith asked.

"I never thought of it that way." Mike said with surprise. "I don't look at the good numbers. I just try to avoid the high ones. Honestly, I don't know what makes them good or makes them bad."

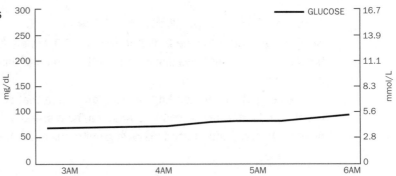

FIGURE 2.8 As Joanna's body prepares to wake, her blood sugars start to increase.

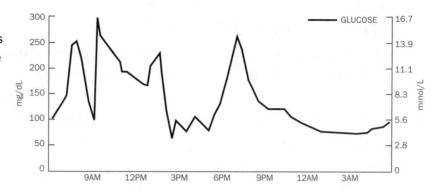

FIGURE 2.9 Here are Joanna's blood sugars over the course of the entire day.

Context Matters

Mike was focused on fixing problems, not preventing them in the first place. And doubling the number of times he checked his sugars hadn't helped. Mike's insurance company did not want to pay for four test strips per day. Dr. Keith had protested that the extra strips were necessary to help Mike identify the cause of his elevated sugar levels. Yet, doing it this way hadn't helped. Mike's diary was full of numbers, but the numbers were only part of the story.

This gap is common, even though it's obvious that having a list of numbers without the corresponding times and events makes it impossible to know what happened. Did a fight with a friend cause a high sugar or was it the slice of cheesecake? Did exercising cause the low blood sugar or too much medication before lunch? Mike needed to gather details to close this gap and understand the impact of his actions on blood sugars.

Note the Good Moments

Asking Mike to come back in three months hadn't helped much, either. Dr. Keith could have gathered the same information in a week by checking Mike's sugars 28 times, instead of 336.

Ask yourself: are you focusing on the highs and lows while ignoring the good numbers you want? How did those periods of normal blood sugars happen? What caused them to go out of that range? Can you make those periods last longer? When you approach it this way, you will be able to make those "good" sugars happen again and again.

THE PROBLEM WITH HEALTH CARE

The frustrating thing about health care in the U.S. and many other countries is that it will only pay to solve a crisis. Are your blood sugars so high you need to be hospitalized? The system will pay. Do you have an infection? The system will pay. Are you waking up feeling lousy every morning? Sorry. The health care system isn't designed to make you feel good, it's designed to avoid expensive catastrophes. It is designed to fix things using drugs and surgery.

Most doctors would love to help their patients manage chronic conditions. Until recently, they could not depend on payment for the types of solutions we discuss in this book, so they rarely made the time. The good news is this dynamic is changing. People throughout the health care system understand that it's "broken," and there are lots of ideas about how to fix it. Yet, such a complex and unwieldy system takes a long time to adapt and change effectively. If you choose to wait for changes, you may be waiting a long time.

Chapter 3

Take Charge
with Knowledge

O ne of the keys to making diabetes easier to manage is to become familiar with
the tools in your toolkit. These tools help to measure your blood sugars and
influence them to go up or down. You may be surprised at some tools that
you've had all along but haven't been using. Getting a solid understanding of the tools
may take a little time. Many books cover this information in a hundred pages or more.
We have focused on the information you can use to take action.

WAYS TO MEASURE BLOOD SUGAR
We talk a lot about blood sugar in this book. Let's step back and look at how to
measure it.

Blood Glucose Meters
Your blood glucose meter is one of the most important tools for monitoring
your diabetes.[14] You must follow the instructions for calibrating (if necessary) and
using your meter. You need to be able to trust that the results you are getting
are accurate.

The technology may be sophisticated, but the idea is simple. Your meter takes a
drop of blood and looks at how much sugar is in that drop. In the United States, this is
measured in milligrams of sugar per deciliter of blood. It's abbreviated as mg/dL or

just mg for short. Outside of the United States, measurements are based on millimoles per liter of blood, abbreviated as mmol/L.

Before you check your blood sugar, wash your hands. This is especially important if you've touched food recently. You want to measure the sugar in your blood, not the jelly left on your fingertips. If you have an incorrect high blood sugar reading because of something on your fingers and take a medication like insulin, it can result in a severe and dangerous low blood sugar. You don't need to use alcohol swabs first. This will dry out your skin over time and can sting when you use the lancet.

Where you check your blood sugars also matters. Some meters support checking blood from places other than your finger, such as your arm. These numbers will lag behind the numbers you get from your fingers. For example, if your blood sugar dropped from 75 mg/dL to 55 mg/dL (4.2 mmol/L to 3.1 mmol/L) over the last fifteen minutes, checking in your arm may give you a result of 70 mg/dL (3.9 mmol/L) while checking with your finger will give you the more current 55 mg/dL (3.1 mmol/L). So if you're checking for low blood sugars, always use your fingers to get the most accurate results.

Always make sure that you have enough blood to fill the test strip. Using too little blood is a major cause of incorrect meter readings.

You must be careful to store test strips properly. If they get too hot, too cold, or exposed to moisture, they can become inaccurate. You need to be careful about leaving them in a car on a sunny day or keeping the container open for too long.

Protecting your test strips is especially important if you are taking blood-sugar lowering medication based on your blood sugars.

Lab-Drawn Blood Sugar Test

Sometimes, your health care provider will draw a vial of blood from your vein and check the blood sugar in a lab. This type of test is more accurate because it uses a larger volume of blood and much more expensive equipment. This type of blood sugar test is a routine part of a typical doctor's appointment for someone with diabetes.

The number you get from a lab-drawn blood sugar will be a little different than what your meter says. You meter measures the amount of sugar in your whole blood. The test in the lab begins by removing the red blood cells and only looking at the sugar in the liquid that remains.

Continuous Glucose Meters

Continuous glucose meters (CGMs) track changes in the sugar in the fluid under your skin, called interstitial fluid, every five minutes. To use it, you place a sensor the size of a matchbook on top of your skin. This sensor includes a tiny piece of plastic that goes just a few millimeters under your skin. Sensors are typically approved to be worn for up to a week and then removed, though many people wear them for up to two weeks before the body's natural healing processes start to block the sensor under your skin and prevent it from working.

When there is a change in the amount of sugar in your blood, it may take up to 15 minutes for the amount of sugar in your interstitial fluid to change to the same level.

Currently, CGMs are not accurate enough to fully replace blood glucose meters. You should use a blood glucose meter to check your blood sugar prior to taking an injection of insulin or treating a low reading on a CGM.

A1c: Average Blood Sugars

One of the most common measures of blood sugars over time is called a Hemoglobin A1c, typically shortened to A1c or HbA1c. This gives you an estimate of your blood sugars over the last few months.

Here's how it works. When there is sugar in your blood, some of it bonds with your red blood cells. These red blood cells have a lifespan of about three months, so we can get an approximation of your average blood sugars. People commonly say that the A1c measures your blood sugars over the last three months, but about ninety percent of the A1c is determined during the last 60 days.

For someone without diabetes, a normal A1c is below 5.7%. What is the ideal target for someone with diabetes? That is a balancing act. The closer you get to the

A1CS AND AVERAGE BLOOD SUGARS

Here is a table showing the relationship between your A1c and average blood sugars. Your average blood sugars are often abbreviated as eAG, which is short for "estimated average glucose." In the United States, we use mg/dL to measure blood sugars (the middle column). In much of the rest of the world, we measure in mmol/L (the right column).

A1c (%)	Estimated Average Glucose (mg/dL) (United States)	Estimated Average Glucose (mmol/l) (Most Non-U.S. Countries)
5	97	5.4
6	126	7.0
7	154	8.6
8	183	10.2
9	212	11.8
10	240	13.3
11	269	14.9
12	298	16.6

normal range, the more your risk of long-term complications is reduced. However, medications that lower blood sugars increase the risk of severe low blood sugars as you get closer to the normal range, particularly in elderly patients.

Various organizations recommend different targets, typically between 6.5% and 7% unless there are other considerations (e.g., for the elderly or children).[15]

Even if people have A1cs below 6.5%, there may still be risk of complications in the eyes, kidneys, and nerves. A portion of that risk is genetic.

Work your with your doctor to identify an A1c target that makes sense for you.

WHEN TO CHECK FOR KETONES

Ketones can appear when you have high blood sugar or low blood sugar. Their presence in the urine or blood indicates that your cells are starving for energy from a sugar source. Perhaps the sugar levels in the blood are too low, or there's no insulin to bring sugar into the cells.

In these settings, increased ketones are a normal response. However, if high blood sugar causes too many ketones to build up in your blood, blood becomes acidic. Nausea, vomiting, dehydration, coma, and death may occur. Prior to the discovery of insulin, this was the typical cause of death in people with type 1 diabetes.

People with type 1 diabetes should always have easy access to (unexpired!) ketone sticks. If you have type 1 or type 2 and suspect you may be having low blood sugars while sleeping, you can check for ketones in the morning. Their presence is a strong hint that you have had a low blood sugar overnight. These sticks are easy to use. Just apply a small amount of urine to the stick and it changes color based on the presence of ketones.

Hydrate to Remove Ketones

If your ketones are caused by high blood sugars, call your doctor. The typical treatment when sugars are high is insulin to get your levels back into the normal range. This turns off the creation of more ketones by enabling sugar from your bloodstream to move into starving cells. Treatment also includes taking fluids, either by drinking or intravenous injection, to remove ketones from your blood through your kidneys. Frequently, people with ketones in their blood are dehydrated. Ketones can occur especially quickly if you are dehydrated from flu, food poisoning, or other illness.

As long as you can drink fluids, there is a chance to reverse the problem by taking insulin for the high sugar and drinking fluids which contain a balance of electrolytes, like potassium. Time is essential here if you want to avoid a trip to the hospital. If ketones in the urine are present in moderate amounts or more and you are vomiting and cannot drink fluids, you'll need intravenous liquids to turn the situation around. The sooner you get to the hospital, the more likely it will be that you'll be home within a day—as long as another illness like pneumonia or flu did not cause the problem.

Dangerous Ketones in Type 2 Diabetes

While ketones are created most often in people with type 1 diabetes, there is one situation where those with type 2 diabetes may accumulate ketones and be in life-threatening danger. Elderly people with a long history of type 2 diabetes who are not obese or overweight may lose their ability to make insulin when they are ill. Ketone measurement in the urine can be helpful for these people to determine if cells are starving in their body. If so, seek urgent medical care.

YOU *CAN* INFLUENCE YOUR BLOOD SUGARS

Let's return to our premise that you are the person best able to understand your body's needs. A book can't tell you how much insulin or oral medication to take, the optimal settings for an insulin pump, or the most appropriate diet for your goals. This is your responsibility, in consultation with your doctor, nurse, or a registered dietitian (R.D.) who is a certified diabetes educator (CDE).

We hope you'll feel empowered to lead a discussion about whether a medication that has been prescribed for you is the right choice. Go ahead, ask about the risks, side effects, and benefits of other options, including increasing your activity levels or adjusting your diet. People with type 2 diabetes are usually producing more insulin than they realize. The right mix of exercise, food choices, and medications can be very influential in decreasing the amount of medication required.

Many people with type 1 diabetes also produce small amounts of insulin. There are medications that may help augment this natural production. This is a new concept in diabetes research, and worth talking about with your doctor. You might ask for a C-Peptide test to help determine if your body is producing insulin or not, even with a diagnosis of type 1 diabetes.

FOOD FUNDAMENTALS

Food is one of the major blood sugar-increasing factors that is in your control. Hundreds of books have been written about what should be in a "diabetes diet."

Of course, there is no such thing as a diabetes diet. If there were, would apple pie be part of it? You might think a slice has too many carbohydrates. But what about a few bites? What if you balance it out with exercise or insulin? What about eating some pie to prop up your blood sugars and prevent a low after a long workout?

The right diet is one that works for you. In this section, we will look at the basic facts about food and blood sugars so that you can predict the impact of food choices on your sugar levels. We will show how to use this information to make office visits with your doctor, nurse, Certified Diabetes Educator, or dietitian more useful for you.

Counting Carbohydrates

Counting carbohydrates is one of the key things that people who are successful at managing diabetes do. The idea is to add up the total amount of carbohydrates in each meal and snack and keep track of it. You can learn how many carbohydrates your body can process in a given meal and over the course of a whole day. You can learn how many carbohydrates your medications, especially insulin, can handle. People with success find a sweet spot where, if they avoid eating more carbohydrates than that, their diabetes is easier to manage.

Carbohydrates are digested into sugar and absorbed into your bloodstream. Focusing exclusively on sugars rather than on total carbohydrates is a common mistake that newly diagnosed people often make. For example, many will eat a sugar-free cookie that's loaded with carbohydrates and be surprised when their blood sugars skyrocket.

The total carbohydrate count on a nutritional label includes fiber. There is some debate about whether fiber needs to be considered. Research suggests that if you eat a meal high in fiber (more than five grams), it will slow down the absorption of sugar into your bloodstream and may lead to lower sugar levels after a meal. A talk with your dietitian about fiber in your diet may be helpful to decide when to take fiber consumption into account when calculating how many carbohydrates you eat.

You don't need to do math at every meal for the rest of your life. Perfect is the enemy of good here. Be good enough to be successful.

Protein, a Safe Choice

In relation to blood sugars, protein typically has a small impact. When protein is digested, your body can use it to manufacture sugar if it needs it. For those on a low-carb diet, meals high in protein can provide sugar for your body. If your blood sugars are higher than normal, your body will also store protein building blocks for making sugar (called glycogen) for later. We recommend checking your blood sugar before and after a few meals high in protein to see its impact on you. If you have kidney issues, please talk to your doctor about how much protein you can safely include in your diet.

Fat, Not so Bad

Fat has no direct impact on blood sugars. In fact, for those with insulin resistance such as type 2 diabetes, it can help. Fat slows down digestion, giving your body more time to process sugar using natural or injected insulin or medications that stimulate insulin production.

However, if you combine fat with a lot of carbs, this slowdown can cause problems. As many people taking blood sugar-lowering medications quickly discover, it is notoriously hard to figure out how much medication to take for a slice of pizza. Pizza is basically a mix of fat and carbs. The fat can slow down the absorption of the carbohydrates too much and the medication can stop working before the pizza is fully digested. This can lead to low blood sugars shortly after eating or high blood sugars many hours after the meal.

Fat also has an impact on how food feels and tastes in your mouth. (That's one reason why pizza is so popular.) It can increase your appetite. If one of your goals is weight loss, a diet too high in fat can sometimes be an obstacle.

Keep a Food Diary

Food diaries are very important, and so often they fall by the wayside. A valuable tool in the doctor-patient relationship, food diaries bring focus to what can easily be an amorphous discussion during an office visit. This is an opportunity for people with diabetes to get the guidance they need to move forward in their self-care. Yet, food diaries can be time-consuming and frustrating if they don't provide useful information.

To start a food diary, focus on your favorite, frequent meals. Don't try to record everything. You may have questions about a meal where high, or low, sugar levels occur afterwards. You can take this information to your dietitian to discuss. Talk about the role of carbohydrates, fats, and proteins in more detail and how you can use the information in the diary to lower your post-meal sugars. Your appointments will be far more productive! You may also want to bring nutritional information for any of the packaged, fast food, or restaurant items that you frequently eat.

It's good to share the outcome of visits to a dietitian or diabetes educator with your doctor or nurse, so they can support you moving forward in your diabetes self-care. It may bring more focus to the problems you are finding difficult to manage.

JUST GET PHYSICAL!

If you could put the benefits of exercise in a pill and sell it, it would be the greatest blockbuster in the history of medicine. Physical activity is one of the most effective tools for improving your blood sugars.

People who are frequently active need less medication. Exercise reduces insulin requirements, facilitates weight loss, and improves sleep. It strengthens your whole body, especially the cardiovascular system. This last benefit is especially important because heart disease is the leading cause of death for people with diabetes.

Consistency matters. If you do a little bit of exercise every day, even just 20 minutes of brisk walking, it has benefits that last.

Light to Moderate Physical Activity

When your body moves, it processes sugar. The more you move, the more sugar it processes. (Intense physical activity works differently. We'll talk about that next.)

In the Big Blue Test, designed by a nonprofit organization on whose advisory board author David Edelman sits, participants do 14 minutes of physical movement—dancing, walking, hula hooping, anything—and share the results online at www.bigbluetest.org. In a 2012 study, the average participant saw their blood sugars drop over 20 percent in just 20 minutes.[16] And exercise is free! Not bad, right? Physical activity, both light and strenuous, can continue to lower your blood sugar for a long time after you stop moving. In one study, participants who exercised were at a greater risk of low blood sugar for a full 48 hours.

Intense Physical Activity

If you push your body's limits while exercising, it can increase your blood sugars. When Olympic swimmer Gary Hall swims one length of the pool at full speed, his blood sugars can double from 150 mg/dL to 300 mg/dL (8.3 mmol/L to 16.7 mmol/L). Yet, when Gary slows down and swims two lengths at less than sprinting speed, his blood sugars lower from 150 mg/dL (8.3 mmol/L to) to about 90 mg/dL (5 mmol/L).

Most of the time, exercise will lower your blood sugar. But if you're pushing your limits, be aware that it may go up. If you frequently go for a walk and find your blood sugars go up, this may be a sign that your body is under stress. If there was no pain or shortness of breath with your walk, the increased sugar during the walk may be an early indicator of heart disease. Please talk to your doctor about taking a cardiac (heart) stress test if this happens to you. See the Take a Walk diary in the Appendix.

WHERE DO BLOOD SUGARS COME FROM?

Sugar gets into your bloodstream in multiple ways, not just from the food that you eat. For example, stress can cause your liver to release sugar.

Intestines

When food is absorbed in your intestines, carbohydrates are converted to sugar and enter your bloodstream. Your intestines begin making hormones that cause your body to release insulin (stored in your pancreas) before the food is absorbed. If you take insulin, the amount you take to cover your meals is an attempt to mimic this process in your body.

Liver

Your liver can make sugar from protein or store it for later use as something called glycogen. The process of turning protein into sugar is called gluconeogenesis and takes about 25 minutes.

The liver releases stored sugar instantly when you experience low blood sugar, although this process doesn't always work well enough in people with diabetes to prevent or adequately treat them. This is an excellent self-defense mechanism to protect your brain and the rest of you.

WHERE DOES SUGAR GO?
Your Brain

All day, every day, a consistent amount of sugar feeds the brains of all people with or without diabetes. The brain doesn't require insulin to access sugar from the blood stream. In people with low blood sugar, the brain is starved of fuel—a devastating experience. Thankfully, a number of studies have shown that blood sugars as low as 40 mg/dL (2.2 mmol/L) are not associated with long-term damage to the brain.[15, 17]

Muscles

Your muscles use the vast majority of your blood sugar. When you walk around the block and your blood sugars fall, it is becoming fuel for your muscles. The muscles

continued on next page

between your shoulders and your knees use 85 percent of the sugar from your blood stream.

Fat Cells

If your body has excess sugar, it goes to your liver, where it can be stored as excess fat. Having extra insulin in your blood for long periods of time causes your body to lock the fat cells and prevent them from being used as fuel. This is why weight loss is difficult in people with diabetes; the condition is associated with weight gain and sustained obesity.

There is even substantial debate about what comes first, the weight gain leading to diabetes or undiagnosed diabetes causing the weight gain. Later in the book, we'll look at the impact of insulin on weight gain.

Kidneys

When there is too much sugar in your blood (above 180 mg/dL [10 mmol/L] in most people), your kidneys will divert some of it out of the body through your urine.

MANAGE YOUR MEDICATIONS

It's a good idea to talk with your health care team to understand exactly how your medications work, as well as their benefits and risks. Work with the team to determine when to take the medications and how much to take. As the leader of your health care team, it is critical that you know what you are taking and why. Don't outsource this understanding to your doctor. This is an important area for you to take charge.

For medications that lower blood sugars, here are four important questions to ask:

- How soon does it start to lower sugar levels?
- Does it work evenly or is there a period of time when the sugar-lowering effect will be stronger?

- How long does it last?
- How might this medicine hurt me, and what makes it more likely that it will?

It's also important to understand when you should change your medications, especially if your schedule changes. Your doctor won't be there when you wake up three hours later on the weekend or when you travel for vacation, to visit family, or for work. Answers to all of these questions can also be found (for any FDA approved medication) by putting the name of the medicine into your internet browser and adding the letters "PI," for prescribing information.

Although there are many different combinations of medication, there are universal starting points for people with type 1 and type 2 diabetes.[18, 19]

Insulin for Type 1 Diabetes

Everyone with type 1 diabetes requires insulin, by injection, pump, or inhaler. Insulin is one of the body's essential hormones; it unlocks cell doors so sugar can power your body's organs. It also allows the body to store extra sugar as fat for later use. If your body does not produce enough insulin, it can't get enough of the sugar from your blood into your muscles or fat cells. The sugar builds up in the blood and leads to the adverse side effects of diabetes.

The primary side effect of insulin is low blood sugars, which we talk about in great depth throughout the book. When taking insulin, learning how to take the right amount is critically important. Please err on the side of safety and take too little rather than too much insulin when you are in doubt. You can always add more, but you can't remove it once you take it.

Choosing the Right Type 2 Diabetes Treatment

Eating well, increasing your activity, and healthy living are the first-line treatments in managing type 2 diabetes. If you cannot reach your target blood sugars without medication, clinical guidelines recommend starting with an effective and well-tolerated drug called metformin and going from there.

THE MIRACLE OF INSULIN

The discovery of insulin is one of the pivotal moments in the history of medicine. Prior to 1922, diabetes was always fatal in people who had what was then called juvenile diabetes. During the 1910s, the most effective treatment was a starvation diet that could prolong life for up to three years. *The Lancet* published this account in 2011:

[She] was an 11-year-old girl who, in 1919, was diagnosed with what we now call type 1 diabetes, or insulin-dependent diabetes mellitus. Known at the time as "acute" diabetes, it was a death sentence; few people lived more than a few months after diagnosis. But this young girl, Elizabeth Evans Hughes, the daughter of a politically powerful American family, was given the latest treatment available.

The principle behind [Frederick] Allen's diet was simple: patients should only consume as much food as their bodies could efficiently metabolize, however little that was. Allen began treatment by having his patients eat nothing and then slowly added carbohydrates. When sugar appeared in the blood, a patient's tolerance level was established; he or she could now eat only enough to stay below it.

Early death was still inevitable but Allen believed that if patients adhered to his diet they could extend their lives, relieve the distress of otherwise inevitable organ failure, and feel some sense of control over their lives.

For people with "acute" diabetes, tolerance levels were extremely low. Elizabeth, for example, was only allowed to eat about 800 or fewer calories a day with usually one fasting day during each week when she could consume perhaps only 250 calories or nothing at all if a trace of sugar had shown in her daily urine test.

Of course, this was not enough to sustain life.

Elizabeth and other patients on Allen's diet wasted away, falling prey to a variety of infections to which they had no resistance. Not surprisingly, few people were able to stay on this diet, even if they had the desire to do so. But Elizabeth managed to stick rigidly to it and her story has a happy ending. She kept herself alive long enough to become one of the first recipients of insulin when it was first used in clinical trials for human beings in 1922.

If you are unable to achieve your target A1c, typically 6.5%, with lifestyle changes and other medications, then it is important to consider insulin. Diabetes is a progressive condition, and achieving target blood sugars can bring emerging complications to a halt. Early insulin use is far preferable to trying other approaches that aren't working for years and years. Not taking insulin when other agents fail can leave you at higher risk for complications, both now and in the future, and make diabetes increasingly difficult to manage day-to-day.

Natural Insulin Therapy

When produced naturally by beta cells in your pancreas, insulin goes directly into your blood stream based on how much sugar is in the blood. (It's a little more complicated than that, but this is basically true.) Naturally produced insulin works very quickly. It lasts for under two hours, compared to the four-to-six hours that "rapid-acting" insulins last. This means it's more difficult for you to match your body's needs with injected insulin than it is for a fully functioning pancreas. When you get things working well, it's a moment to be proud.

In people with long-time type 2 diabetes and in some with type 1, the body may still be producing insulin. Importantly, these tiny amounts are thought to have a major impact on preventing diabetes complications. Yet, these small amounts are typically not enough to meet the person's needs.

In anyone whose sugars have been high for a long time, starting on insulin therapy is especially beneficial. As your blood sugars go back to their normal range, some of your body's systems will begin to function more effectively. Systems that were maxed out and unresponsive will begin to take over some of the work of balancing your blood sugars.

Daily Basal and Bolus Insulin Requirements

In people without diabetes, the body delivers a constantly varying supply of insulin to match the body's basic needs. People with diabetes must manage that process. To be successful, it's important to understand your body's two different insulin needs.

The first is for "basal" insulin. This is the steady supply of insulin that powers your brain, resting muscles, and other organs. This varies little throughout the day; it's fairly consistent but your needs can go up if your body is under stress from illness, injury, or chronic pain from nerve damage (diabetic neuropathy). Without the natural production of basal insulin, even if you don't eat any food, your blood sugars will rise throughout the day as your liver releases sugar to power your basic needs.

There are a few ways to get basal insulin. One is by injecting long-acting insulin. Another is with multiple injections of faster and shorter-acting insulin. The last is by using an insulin pump that continuously delivers small amounts of fast-acting insulin throughout the day, mimicking the way the body naturally performs.

The second need is for "bolus insulin" to cover short-term spikes in blood sugars. This happens when you eat a meal containing carbohydrates or experience a stressful situation, which causes your liver to release significant amounts of sugar. To process that sugar, you need a larger amount of insulin over a shorter period of time. This is also sometimes called a "food bolus," "meal bolus," or "correction dose."

If you are prescribed two types of insulin, one is typically for covering your basal needs and the other for bolus needs. This is called basal-bolus therapy.

Tips for Injecting Insulin

Insulin should be injected under your skin and not into muscle. If you inject insulin into muscle, it is not only painful, but acts extremely quickly and can cause severe low blood sugars. The insulin stays active in your body for far less time than when it's taken under the skin.

Insulin can also act more quickly if taken in your limbs, such as in your thigh instead of your abdomen. This is especially true if you are being physically active. Studies have shown it's about 15% more potent.[20]

Here are some tips for injecting insulin:

- When injecting in your arms, use the fatty tissue in the back of the arm near your shoulder.
- When injecting into your buttocks, use the fatty tissue by your hip or in the back where a wallet would go.
- Make sure injections are at least an inch apart to give your body time to heal.
- Avoid injecting anywhere you have scar tissue, broken vessels, or varicose veins.
- To speed up absorption, you can massage the area of the injection or apply heat. On the other hand, cold slows down insulin.
- Dry skin can increase your rate of insulin absorption. You may notice your insulin needs change when you turn on the heat in winter climates.
- Larger doses of insulin take longer to start working and last longer.
- If you are using an insulin pen, leave the tip in for a few moments to ensure that none of the insulin leaks out.

TYPES OF INSULIN

Your doctor may prescribe you different types of insulin, and you need to know why he is giving you a particular type. Your pharmacist or a CDE can tell you if it is basal or bolus insulin, when it should start to work, when it should peak, and when it should stop working.

It is very important to understand the dangers of any insulin you are taking. In a discussion about medical errors and adverse events called "To Err is Human," the Institute of Medicine in 1999 identified insulin as one of the most worrisome medications used.[21] There is a very small difference between the perfect, helpful dose of insulin and an overdose. The limitations and dangers are spelled out in the prescribing information (PI) about each insulin product, which is available online. There are wide variations in how insulin acts in different people; however, it is usually consistent in each individual if injected properly.

Long-Acting Insulin

Long-acting insulins meet your body's ongoing insulin needs. They are not meant to cover spikes in blood sugars caused by a meal. They do not lower a high blood sugar quickly. This class of insulins first became available in 2000 with the approval of Lantus (glargine) in the United States. It was soon followed by Levemir (detemir).

These insulins begin to act shortly after insertion. However, their ability to lower sugar slowly increases until they reach a consistent level after about four to six hours. A single daily injection under your skin may last 20 to 28 hours. Long-acting insulins cannot perfectly match your body's basal insulin needs, which tend to change throughout the day and night.

Hormone rhythms cause your liver to release sugar for energy when your body prepares to wake up from sleep. In the late afternoon, your basal needs tend to fall, which could increase your risk of low blood sugars during this part of the day. This means that you may need more insulin in the morning and lower amounts in the afternoon for the same carbohydrate intake.

Always be sure to inject under the skin and not into muscle when using long acting insulins. If you are thin, elderly, or caring for someone else, be especially alert.

Rapid-Acting Insulin

Rapid-acting insulins, also called fast-acting, cover meal-time insulin needs or lower high blood sugars. This class of insulin came with the 1996 approval of Humalog (lispro). It was soon joined by Novolog (aspart) and later by Apidra (glulisine).

When given below the skin, these insulins start working in 10 to 30 minutes, usually peak in 60 to 90 minutes, and last under 5 hours. These are the fastest-acting insulins available, although research is underway to make them faster and last for a shorter amount of time than their typical four hours. There is wide variation in how insulins work among people. So these times should be considered guidelines and not hard facts.

If you have type 2 diabetes and your body is not producing enough insulin, you will often be prescribed a rapid-acting insulin to cover your post-meal high blood sugars. Everyone with type 1 diabetes should be taking a rapid-acting insulin, either through injections or an insulin pump.

Intermediate-Acting Insulin

This class of insulin takes an hour or two to start and lasts for 4 to 12 hours. It is commonly called NPH (neutral protamine Hagedorn) or by the names Humulin N, Novolin N, Novolin NPH, NPH Iletin II, and isophane insulin. NPH has greater peaks than other insulins. If you take it at night, you are at a higher risk of low blood sugars. If you have a bad reaction to other insulins, your doctor may prescribe it. It is also less expensive than most other insulins.

Regular or Short-Acting Insulin

Regular insulin is sold under the brand names Humulin and Novolin. Contrary to the name, there is nothing particularly "regular" about it. It acts more quickly than the intermediate-acting insulins and less quickly than rapid-acting insulins. It lasts 4 to 12 hours, making it unpredictable.

Mixed Insulin

Mixed insulins are designed to reduce the number of injections required to manage sugar levels. If you have type 2 diabetes and you are taking insulin injections three or more times per day, then mixed insulin may reduce your injection frequency to once or twice daily. That's the good news.

The challenge with mixed insulins is that they contain two different types of insulins. So instead of dealing with two insulins that you can adjust independently, you are locked into a fixed ratio. It can be challenging to match a mixed insulin to your body's actual insulin needs.

All of the mixed insulins contain intermediate-acting insulin (NPH). They also contain either a regular, short-acting insulin or a rapid-acting insulin. It is very important to understand the ratio of the insulins you are taking, so don't switch to a different formulation without talking to your doctor.

Mixed insulins may be appropriate if your body is still producing and using insulin normally, but not sufficiently to control sugar levels. If you have sustained high blood sugars or large swings, then it is probably not for you. It is not for people with type 1 diabetes.

Inhaled Insulin

Inhaled insulin is a newly available option. It is only available as a substitute for rapid-acting insulin, not long-acting insulin. The key benefit is that it does not require an injection. The primary side effects are shortness of breath and coughing. Research on their long-term effects is limited.

Insulin Pens

Insulin pens are pre-filled cartridges of insulin that easily fit in your pocket. They allow you to more easily adjust your insulin dose with less chance of error. They also use smaller needles than insulin syringes, which reduces the risk that you will inject insulin into your muscle and makes them less painful. Pens are available for both long-acting and rapid-acting insulins.

Insulin Pumps

Insulin pumps can be useful for those who want more precise control over their insulin delivery and are willing to program it. Insulin pumps deliver a steady supply of rapid-acting insulin through a tiny plastic tube (called a "canula") under your skin. Instead of multiple daily injections, you simply insert a new infusion set every three or so days.

You can program an insulin pump to deliver a small amount of insulin through-out the day to match your basal insulin needs. You can also tell it to give you larger doses of insulin to match a meal or correct a high blood sugar. For example, when your insulin needs are higher in the morning, it can be programmed to deliver more insulin. When you are snacking at a party all afternoon, you can tell it to deliver your meal-time bolus over a number of hours instead of all at once. Such flexibility is very difficult to accomplish with insulin injections.

Insulin pumps do not require surgery to install, but they can be expensive. They also require more skill and understanding to set up and use because you have to manage the pump and the diabetes together. However, for people with type 1 diabetes, insulin pumps can make thriving with diabetes more achievable than using injections.

THE TEMPERAMENTAL PUMP

Insulin pumps are not an artificial pancreas—you have to tell them what to do. If an insulin pump fails, it can lead to very high blood sugars and ketoacidosis. There is also a minor risk of infection where the insulin is delivered under your skin if the infusion sites—where the insulin goes into the body—are not monitored.

In spite of the risks, if you are taking multiple daily injections of insulin, we recommend considering an insulin pump. Current and aspiring insulin pumpers can use the two books below to learn how to get the most out of their pumps. Links to both books are available at www.dthrive.com/pumps.

- *Pumping Insulin: Everything You Need to Succeed on an Insulin Pump* by John Walsh, P.A., and Ruth Roberts, M.A. (2012).
- *Insulin Pumps and Continuous Glucose Monitoring: A User's Guide to Effective Diabetes Management* by Francine R. Kaufman (2012).

THE PROMISE OF AN ARTIFICIAL PANCREAS

You may have heard about the "artificial pancreas" or "bionic pancreas." This refers to a system that continuously monitors your blood sugars and automatically adjusts the amount of insulin to manage them. Some systems also pump glucagon to raise blood sugars when needed.

As we write this, there are no fully automated systems available outside of clinical trials. The first steps, however, are in place. Medtronic has an insulin pump that shuts off insulin delivery if the continuous glucose sensors detect that you will soon have a low blood sugar.

There are also multiple studies on implantable devices that contain insulin-producing cells. These devices function as small, self-contained pancreases and automatically manage your blood sugars. As of publication, all of these devices are in early stages of human testing and will require many more years (and possibly decades) of work before they are commercially available.

There has been enormous progress in the effectiveness of these systems. In some studies, people have seen blood sugars significantly closer to the normal range while also experiencing fewer low blood sugars.[22] Still, many challenges need to be overcome before they are publicly available.

We are rooting for the researchers investing so much in making these automated diabetes management systems a reality.

NON-INSULIN MEDICATIONS

We don't expect you to memorize all the medications below. The key is to understand how your medications work. Focus on those. In particular, you want to understand the benefits, limitations, and possible side effects.

If you're not achieving your targets, it's worth bringing the list of medications to your doctor to talk about what other options might be appropriate. If you're taking three medications and not achieving your blood sugar goals, something other than your diabetes is wrong, and you may require insulin.

If you take multiple medications, look closely at the risks of low blood sugars and other side effects. Those risks can add up. They may show up as minor problems at first, but minor problems can grow into bigger ones. Be sure to check in with a medical professional if you experience side effects.

A list of the generic and brand names of these medications is located in Appendix B (page 191). Take a moment now to identify the class of medications you are taking.

Metformin

Metformin causes your liver to produce less sugar.[23] Its minor side effects include diarrhea, nausea, bloating, and decreased vitamin B_{12} levels. The diarrhea may be significant. If this is an issue, ask your doctor about changing the form or the time you take metformin. Some people find that taking metformin in the middle of a meal helps, rather than the beginning or end. If you experience stomach issues for more than a week, check with your doctor. A small minority of people simply doesn't tolerate metformin very well.

Sulfonylureas

Sulfonylureas encourage your body to make as much insulin as possible, regardless of how much sugar is in the blood. Consequently, one of the major side effects is low blood sugar, especially when taken with other oral medications or insulin.

Some sulfonylureas remain active in the body for five or six days after the last dose. So if low blood sugars occur, you may need to change your approach for most

RARE, DANGEROUS SIDE EFFECT OF METFORMIN

Metformin has a potentially lethal side effect called lactic acidosis. This often shows up first as excessive fatigue, muscle aches, or kidney problems. It is very uncommon but dangerous, so talk with your doctor to ensure that you understand what to watch out for, especially if you have a history of kidney or chronic heart disease.

of the next week. Hospitalization may be necessary for overdoses. If you have kidney or liver problems, sulfonylureas may add an extra risk of low blood sugars.

TZDs

TZDs cause your muscles to use more sugar. These medications may also cause the liver to produce a little less sugar, making it more difficult for the body to naturally counteract low blood sugars. This is typically only a problem when combined with other blood sugar-lowering medications.

The prescribing information on TZDs includes warnings about using this class of medications in people with heart failure and swollen lower legs and ankles because it increases your risk of fluid accumulation. This is especially true if you have kidney problems. There remains some controversy about the increased risk of heart disease in people who take these medications. While the research is incomplete, the U.S. Food and Drug Administration has concluded that increased risk of heart attacks with TZD use has not been substantiated as of a November 25, 2013 announcement.[24]

GLP-1s

GLP-1s and the similar GLP-1 Receptor Agonists both cause the body to produce more insulin when there is more sugar in the blood and to decrease its glucose lowering action when the sugar levels fall. Because of this, there is a much lower risk of low blood sugars than with sulfonylureas or insulin use. GLP-1s slow down the stomach so that your intestines absorb sugar more slowly. This can also cause you to feel full more quickly and eat less. It's associated with weight loss.

Low blood sugars are rare if you are only taking a GLP-1. However, when combined with insulin or sulfonylureas, GLP-1 use can be associated with low blood sugars.[25] It does this by telling your liver to release less sugar. The most common side effects of GLP-1s are stomach issues such as diarrhea, vomiting, and bloating.

DPP-4 Inhibitors

There is an enzyme in your blood called DPP-4 that can block your helpful GLP-1 hormones. The DPP-4 inhibitors work by stopping the DPP-4 enzymes and giving you the GLP-1 hormones that your body naturally produces more time to work and lower blood sugars. They are about half as effective as GLP-1 receptor agonist medications in lowering your A1c, but have fewer side effects. The side effects are typically the same stomach issues as seen in GLP-1s. If you have lost kidney function, adverse side effects can be amplified. However, this restriction does not apply to linagliptin because linagliptin is not processed by your kidneys.

SGLT-2s

SGLT-2s cause the kidneys to release more sugar in your urine. They do this by preventing your kidneys from putting sugar back into your bloodstream. They do not have any other known impact. In addition to lowering blood sugars, the removal of all of those calories can lead to weight loss. Due to more frequent urination as your body expels that sugar, blood pressure can decrease in some people with hypertension. The major side effect is urinary tract infection and genital infections (mostly, but not exclusively, in women).

Glynides

Glynides act like sulfonylureas by causing your body to make more insulin. They work faster and don't last as long, requiring more frequent doses. They lower blood sugars more rapidly, especially during or after exercising. The most common side effect is low blood sugars.

Alpha-Glucosidase Inhibitor

These reduce the amount of carbohydrates absorbed through your intestines. Importantly, they lower A1c levels by as much as 1%. The biggest side effect is unpleasant flatulence.

STRESS AND WEIGHT MANAGEMENT

Learning to manage stress is an important but under-recognized tool for managing blood sugars.[26] Stress is a general term for a cause of increased demands on your body or mind. It causes your body to release hormones that change how you process blood sugar.

When your body is stressed, either physically or emotionally, it releases stress hormones. This can dump large amounts of sugar into your blood in seconds. In short, it's giving your body all the energy it needs to fight or flee quickly. This can be short-term, like when Joanna was nearly in a car accident, or chronic, if you have pain from nerve damage, depression, or even intense worries about your finances.

The frustrations of managing diabetes can cause even more stress, making it more difficult to manage. Stress can arise out of fear for your safety or long-term health or anger at the impact diabetes is having on your life. Fortunately, these stressors can be reduced through a combination of learning the *Thriving with Diabetes* process and taking care of your emotional wellbeing. If frustration is causing you large amounts of stress, see our discussion on diabetes distress and burnout on page 166, and Thrive for Life on page 133.

Weight Loss and Gain

When you are overweight, your insulin needs increase. Getting to a normal weight can make diabetes significantly easier to manage. Simply put, there are two ways to lose weight: calorie restriction and increased physical activity.

Restricting how many calories you eat is the most effective way to lose weight without surgery—even more so than increasing exercise. The challenge is that people often have a hard time sustaining a lower calorie diet. And it takes a few weeks before the body starts to lose weight. Before this happens, the apparent weight loss has to do with changes in water balance. The fat cells are acclimating to the need for fewer calories during this time period. As you reduce your calorie (and carbohydrate) intake, your insulin needs begin to drop. When they get low enough, the fat cells are unlocked, and your body can turn to them for fuel without producing acidosis with ketones. Your weight begins to burn away. When you are physically active on a regular basis, sugar goes into your muscles more easily. Your insulin needs reduce significantly. Together, this can make it easier for your body to turn to fat for energy.

Insulin, Medications, and Weight Loss

Some medications can make it easier to lose weight; others make it harder. Make sure you talk to your doctor about how any medications you are taking impact your ability to lose weight if that is one of your goals.

Insulin can also have a negative impact on weight loss attempts. When you have extra sugar in your blood and high levels of lipids (fats), insulin increases the size of your fat cells. When you have more insulin in your blood than you need, it prevents your body from releasing that fat. It is biologically impossible to lose weight. If you are taking more than a normal dose of insulin, which is about 20 to 30 units of day for someone between 125 and 150 pounds (57 and 68 kg), this can become a problem. It can also be a problem if you take medication that stimulates extra insulin production.

To lose weight, you must reduce your body's need for insulin. You can adopt a regular exercise program to make your body more sensitive to insulin. You can eat a lower carbohydrate diet so that your body needs to process less sugar. It could also mean changing medications that you are on.

For those injecting insulin, issues with weight loss are more frequent with pre-meal regular insulin. It is less common with rapidly acting insulins that are popular today because they are associated with lower after-meal sugar levels.

If you are looking to lose weight, it is especially important to minimize blood sugar swings to limit blood sugar roller coasters. Whenever you have a lot of sugar and insulin in your body, it is difficult to lose weight.

Weight Loss Surgery

Weight loss surgery has been surprisingly effective at improving or even reversing type 2 diabetes. In almost eight percent of cases, patients no longer need diabetes medications and achieve normal blood sugars. The effects are almost immediate. The average weight loss is over 60 percent of the excess weight.[27]

There are multiple types of weight loss surgery. Some are permanent and some can be reversed. Some are more complex than others. This is a viable option for many, but there are side effects to consider. In addition to the normal risks of surgery, the short-term side effects are getting full faster, abdominal cramping, and increased risk of low blood sugars, especially if you do not reduce your blood sugar-lowering medication after surgery. Long-term risks may include nutritional deficiencies and osteoporosis. As with all surgeries, make sure that you fully understand the risks associated.

PART 2

THE 4-STEP ACTION PLAN

"The treatment of a patient with diabetes lasts a long time. Treatment [should be] carried on with as little interference with the daily routine as possible."

—Dr. Elliott Joslin

Chapter 4

Step 1: Lower the Highs

A s diabetes develops, your blood sugars slowly start to rise. In taking action, the first step is to lower high blood sugars. However, once your blood sugars near the normal range, you become at risk for low blood sugars. Thus, diabetes becomes a balancing act: keeping blood sugars low enough to avoid long-term complications, but high enough to avoid the dangers of low blood sugars.

KEEP SUGAR TRAFFIC MOVING TO YOUR CELLS

Let's imagine your blood vessels are highways. Each bit of sugar is a car traveling down a highway to get to its exit—a cell that needs sugar for energy. In someone without diabetes, the traffic is light. After a meal, it may get busier, but the car still gets to its exit and makes it home on time.

In someone with diabetes, exit ramps get clogged as the highway drops from four lanes to one. In people who produce no insulin whatsoever, the exit ramps shut down almost completely. This causes all the blood sugar traffic to back up in the blood-stream, resulting in high blood sugars.

When blood sugars rise above 200 mg/dL (11.1 mmol/L), traffic gets so backed up that simply re-opening the exits doesn't work very well. Traffic keeps coming faster than cars can get off the road. The traffic jam gets even worse if your body is under stress. Stress, whether physical or emotional, tells your body to start dumping even more cars onto the highway. If there's not enough insulin to keep the exit ramps open and too many cars get on the highway, it starts to look like rush hour in Los Angeles.

The thing to understand here is that when your blood sugars are below 200 mg/dL (11.1 mmol/L), the highway system functions far better, and it's easier to fix traffic problems. When sugar levels start to go higher, more aggressive measures are needed to resolve problems.

Your biology is more complicated than this metaphor suggests. There are over a hundred systems in your body which impact how many cars are on the road. When it comes to lowering high blood sugars, perfection is not an option. You can't control these hundred systems any more than a city engineer in Los Angeles can control rush hour. However, you do have a lot of *influence*, like the city engineer who tells people to avoid traveling during rush hour and monitors exits to make sure they stay open. The key skill for influencing traffic patterns is to understand when and why the highways get backed up. This gives you the power to take pre-emptive action by keeping cars off the road or opening extra exit ramps. In this chapter, we will show you how to do both.

THE RULE OF THREES

Learning how to effectively treat and lower a high blood sugar is an important skill. Yet, this is not enough for long-term success. Once you have a high blood sugar, the thing that caused it has already happened. Understanding how to keep sugar levels from rising too much in the first place is a great challenge in managing diabetes. If you don't understand the causes, you'll never be able to effectively influence your sugars. We

KEEP YOUR FOCUS ON YOU!

Different people respond uniquely to foods. When you think about others' experiences, bear in mind this variation. Some people can eat a handful of strawberries with no problem, while others will see their blood sugars go through the roof. At the same time, the strawberry-lover might watch blueberries drive up her blood sugars, while her friend barely registers a bump.

have already covered a wide range of things that cause your blood sugars to go up and down: what you eat, your activity levels, your body's hormonal rhythms, pain, and stress. How can you make the relationship between so many different things simpler to understand and manage on a day-to-day basis without being overwhelmed?

The solution is to use the Rule of Threes. This is an easy strategy for understanding how one thing impacts your blood sugars. As you look at making your diabetes predictable, there is one question you must always ask: how does an event change my blood sugars? The Rule of Threes helps you answer that question. And it's quite simple:

1. Check your blood sugar.
2. Do something.
3. Check your blood sugar again.

Repeat the process on three different days to make sure you get a consistent answer before making up your mind. Now the event has a predictable effect. You can test changes to get the results you want. Rather than looking at everything —which is overwhelming and often useless—you can look at one important thing at a time. Let's take a look at how Martha dealt with this.

A Love for Blueberries

At a youthful 72-years-old, Martha was always pushing her doctor to help her get better at managing her type 2 diabetes.

"I'm always high after breakfast," she exclaimed.

Dr. Franks smiled. "What are you typically eating for breakfast?"

Martha explained that she'd started each day with a bowl of oatmeal and, when they were in season, blueberries, for most of her life. She'd add a little bit of whole milk and, before her diagnosis, a pinch of brown sugar. She had since avoided the pinch of brown sugar.

Her doctor nodded. "Let's do a little experiment. Over the next week, I want you to check your blood sugars before and two hours after breakfast.

On the first three days, eat your oatmeal without blueberries. On the next three days after that, have your blueberries as usual. Give me a call and let me know what happens."

When Martha called back, she needled her doctor. "I just know you are going to tell me to skip my blueberries." She had discovered that blueberries had a surprisingly big impact on her blood sugars. On days without them, her sugars before lunch were actually in her target range.

Dr. Franks reassured her. "I won't take away your blueberries, Martha. Let me share a few different options. We can talk about them, and you can decide what you'd like to do."

....

Like Martha, you can use the Rule of Threes to figure out the impact of breakfast on your blood sugars. If they are too high, you have a few simple options, which we'll discuss further in this chapter.

1. **Eat fewer carbohydrates.** For Martha, that could be a smaller portion of oatmeal, removing the blueberries, or switching to eggs (which have barely one gram of carbs).

2. **Increase activity levels.** Martha could go for a 20-minute walk before or after the meal and measure the impact.

3. **Take more insulin or appropriate medication.** If your doctor has you taking a mealtime dose, he may recommend increasing it in small steps to cover all of the carbohydrates.

When to Check Your Sugars

If you are looking to check at meal time, you could check one to two hours after you eat. It is frequently useful to do both to have a complete picture, although most doctors tend to focus on the two-hour number. When you measure at one hour, you are looking at the highest peak after your meal. At two hours, you are looking at your body's ability to get back to target range. Be thoughtful about what you are measuring. Over time, it becomes less necessary once a meal becomes predictable to you.

For an activity, you will typically check your sugars right after it is done. For the readings to be meaningful, there are a several things to consider:

- If your starting blood sugars are very different, you will get different results. This is especially true if you are starting with a blood sugar below 70 mg/dL (3.9 mmol/L) or over 140 mg/dL (7.8 mmol/L). In these cases, there are other things going on in your body influencing the results that we will talk about later.

- Avoid using the Rule of Threes to identify patterns when your blood sugars are changing rapidly. This can complicate your answers. It's much more effective to do an experiment when you have been lounging around for a few hours than after a two-hour workout. (Unless, of course, you want to measure the impact of a workout!)

- You may discover that doing things at different times of day has different results. For example, people are usually more insulin resistant first thing in the morning than in the late afternoon. So comparing an event that you usually do in the morning with the same activity done in the afternoon will often give you different results.

IDENTIFY CONFOUNDERS

If your body is under constant stress, high blood sugars can be nearly impossible to stabilize. The stress response can increase your resistance to insulin and make lowering sugar levels far more difficult.

We call the things that make blood sugars resistant to lowering "confounders," which means things that cause confusion. Here are some factors that fit into this category:

Illness
- Heart disease
- Lung disease
- Gastrointestinal problems
- Infection
- Other illnesses

Severe Emotional Stress
- Challenging family situations
- Stressful job problems
- Intense financial worries
- Prolonged fear, regret, or anxiety
- Depression

Physical Variables
- Chronic pain
- Exercising beyond your comfort level
- Medication that causes high blood sugars
- Sleep that is frequently interrupted, too short, or skipped entirely
- Frequent low blood sugars

If you don't identify and work on these issues, your blood sugars may remain stubbornly high and unpredictable. Confounders are not always obvious, as Joan's story demonstrates. Hers were hiding in plain sight.

An Unexpected Guest

Since her diagnosis 15 years ago, Joan had hated her diabetes. Nevertheless, she had done everything she could to keep her glucose levels "at goal." She had lived in fear of losing her vision or getting an infection on her feet that might lead to an amputation.

At 34, married with two children, Joan had a great job as a civil engineer that allowed her to be home in the morning when her children left for school and be there in the afternoon when they came home. Every three months, she would visit her endocrinologist. When she saw him last, her hemoglobin A1c was higher than usual, at 7.9%. Her goal for this number had been 6.5%. That meant her average glucose level had been about 180 mg/dL (10 mmol/L) during the previous months.

"What am I doing wrong?" she asked her doctor. "What else can I do?"

As he reviewed her blood sugar diary, her doctor saw that many of the readings were taken in the middle of the night. He asked her why. It turned out that Joan's mother-in-law, Susan, had come to live with Joan and her family for three months. Susan's kitchen had caught fire, making her house unlivable.

Joan disliked her mother-in-law almost as much as she disliked her diabetes. Living with this woman was stressful. Joan had even increased her hours at work to avoid spending time with her mother-in-law. It all added up to a major disruption in Joan's carefully arranged routine of caring for her family and herself.

A big part of Joan's frustration was that her numbers didn't seem that much higher. Her diary showed levels that were lower than 180 mg/dL (10 mmol/L) most of the time. Some levels were over 200 mg/dL (11.1 mmol/L), but not enough to explain the elevated level of A1c. However, a closer look at the diary showed that Joan was not checking her glucose as often as she had previously.

"I just don't have time anymore. Susan is always trying to be helpful, but it drives me crazy. I cannot sleep at night and sometimes, I'm stressing about all of the things I have to do."

Joan's doctor suggested that her elevated glucose levels were due to the stress of having Susan in the house, as well as the change in her schedule and loss of sleep. Since Susan was going back home in two weeks, he recommended that she not make any changes, except going home and getting a good night's sleep.

Three months later, Joan's Hemoglobin A1c was 6.9%. Joan had done nothing "wrong" in caring for her diabetes. Circumstances had changed in Joan's life. If Susan had lived with Joan's family much longer, major adjustments in Joan's diabetes management may have been necessary. As it happened, it all took care of itself.

HOW TO TREAT HIGH BLOOD SUGARS

Once you have the confounders under control, it's time to focus more closely on managing high blood sugars. Please remember to consult your doctor before stopping, starting, or changing your treatment approaches. The process starts by using the Rule of Threes to understand the impact of an event on your blood sugars. You can then use the tools below to lower them to where they need to be.

Change What and When You Eat

One easy way to lower your blood sugars is by changing your food choices. Modest changes in the foods you eat frequently can have a big impact on results.

The most obvious change is to reduce the amount of carbohydrates you are eating. Be very careful to look at total carbohydrates and not just sugar. The total amount is what will cause your blood sugars to rise. One common mistake is to eat a sugar-free cookie loaded with carbohydrates.

The less obvious change is to increase the amount of fat in a meal. Fat slows down digestion, so the sugar will reach your bloodstream more slowly. The time of day that you eat a meal matters, too. If you are more insulin resistant in the morning, then moving a higher carbohydrate meal to later in the day can make it easier for your body to process.

ACCOUNT FOR LENGTHY DIGESTION

If you take insulin, it's important to understand that fast-acting versions last for less than four hours. Meals that are very high in fat and carbohydrates (like pizza) may still be digesting after your insulin stops working. This can lead to dramatic blood sugar spikes many hours after you eat.

Counting Carbs Can be Hard

Some people find counting carbohydrates challenging for a number of reasons. Some are less comfortable working with numbers. Some don't understand what the numbers mean on a nutritional label. Others feel that looking at the contents of food takes the joy out of eating. To those, we suggest that you start slowly and easily. Begin with the meal you eat most frequently. This may be your favorite breakfast or weekday lunch. How many carbohydrates are in that meal?

You could make a particular food predictable with the Rule of Threes without ever knowing the amount of carbohydrates inside. But to make foods predictable, it's useful to understand how many carbohydrates you are eating.

The total carbohydrates number might be on the side of the box it came out of or on a nutritional menu at the restaurant where you eat. If you are preparing the meal from whole ingredients, look at a free website like www.calorieking.com or the *CalorieKing* books by Allan Borushek. There are many other websites and books available with this information. The other way is to write down what you eat (or take a picture on your phone!) and talk to your dietitian about it.

Once you figure out the carbohydrates in one meal, move on to another meal that you frequently eat. This slow-but-steady approach ensures that your skills will grow over time without overwhelming you in the near term. As you slowly practice the Rule of Threes, you will get manageable and actionable knowledge about what changes to make.

In addition to your favorite meals, we recommend starting with simple meals first. Complex meals, like a homemade stew with twenty ingredients, can be more challenging to figure out. In that case, you might want to focus on the ingredients that contain the bulk of carbs to get a reasonable estimate. Ignore the spices and ingredients where you are adding just a pinch. The goal is to be reasonably close, not perfect.

Meals with similar amounts of carbohydrates have a similar impact on your blood sugars. As you get better at identifying how many carbohydrates are in the foods you are eating, you'll get better at predicting how new foods will impact your blood sugars. This can make your life much easier over the long run, even though it takes a little extra work up front.

Adjust Your Activity Levels

Physical activity will lower blood sugars as long as it does not stress your body excessively. This makes sense. Your muscles need to burn sugar to move. The more they move, the more sugar they use, and the less is left in your bloodstream.

Many people do not realize how little activity it takes to improve your blood sugar. Standing burns more sugar than sitting. A twenty-minute walk can drop your blood sugar by 20 percent or more. Moderate, sustained activity, like a 60-minute jog or a game of tennis, can cause your body to process more sugar even 24 hours later.

INSULIN USERS, COUNT THE WHOLE DAY

If you are taking insulin to cover your meals, the carbohydrate count is even more important. Taking inappropriate amounts of insulin can launch a roller coaster of ups and downs. To combat this, figure out how many total carbohydrates you eat during the day. If the number is too high, you will be taking large amounts of insulin and having a hard time managing your blood sugars and your weight. There is significant debate over the minimum number of carbohydrates someone needs to be healthy. This is a good conversation to have with your health care team.

REDUCE YOUR NEED FOR INSULIN!

Did you know that some sugar can enter your muscles without insulin? This is true, and the amount of sugar processed without insulin goes up as your body adapts to more physical activity. This is a major benefit of increasing your level of physical activity over time.

Intense exercise, like a hard sprint or power lifting, can stress the body. Your body senses trouble and floods the bloodstream with sugar to prepare it for action. How much activity is needed to stress the body varies from person to person. This response typically only happens when you are well outside your comfort zone.

If you are not a frequent exerciser and would like to be more active, you have two choices.

The first is to begin gradually. Find a program or routine that you like. If you rarely move, this could be a walk around the block after dinner. Any increase in movement is better than no change at all.

Other people have found success making dramatic life changes. It's like a switch is flipped; they get an enormous amount of energy and apply it towards changing their lives. Sometimes, you just decide it's time and do it.

Research shows that both of these approaches can work. The most important thing is for you to *do something*. But talk to your doctor before starting a major new exercise program to ensure there are no underlying health issues, especially early heart disease, which may not have obvious symptoms.

SUGAR-LOWERING MEDICATIONS

Every medication that lowers blood sugar levels does so in its own way. They take different amounts of time to start working, work at various intensities, and last for varied amounts of time. Some work steadily over long periods, while others have distinct peaks of action. Further, when multiple medications are used together, they can impact each other in unforeseen ways. For more information about how your specific medications work, see page 191.

We can't tell you how much of a medication to take or when to take it, but we can talk about general strategies that your doctor might recommend. The key to success is matching your medication or insulin dosage and timing to your body's needs.

Most doctors follow a well-defined order when prescribing treatment for type 1 or type 2 diabetes. Yet, there is some variability and a number of newer, off-label approaches that are always being tried. Diabetes varies more widely from person to person than most people understand, and this means that one treatment approach is never appropriate for everyone.

It may take your doctor a while to determine the right medications and dosages for you. If you feel like a guinea pig, it's because your doctor is trying to figure out what parts of your body's systems are working and which medications can help best.

Taking medication or insulin is not a sign of failure. Your goal is to manage your blood sugars so you can focus on the important parts of your life.

Non-Insulin Treatments for Type 2 Diabetes

If your doctor recommends a medication, it can be a wake-up call to look closely at your food choices and activity levels for managing diabetes. However, because type 2 diabetes is progressive, there typically comes a time when such lifestyle changes are not enough.

HIGH SUGARS AFTER LIGHT EXERCISE

If light activities increase your blood sugar, it could be a sign of an underlying stressor such as early stage heart disease. Discuss this with your doctor if it happens to you.

Medications for type 2 diabetes, working overnight, are often very effective at improving your waking blood sugars. But they can have a hard time during meals when they need to help your body process all of those carbohydrates over a short period of time. You can use the Rule of Threes to understand how high your blood sugars go after meals and to determine if your medication is working well in combination with your food choices.

When type 2 diabetes cannot be managed by diet and exercise alone, metformin is the go-to drug. It is a safe and effective option. (There are risks to any medication, so please carefully read the product information or label on every medication you are prescribed.) If metformin works for you, it tends to keep working. It is also very affordable.

If your A1c is more than a point above target, medical recommendations suggest using a combination of drugs if necessary. Because each class of drug works on a different part in the body, as we discussed in Chapter 3, they can often work extremely well in combination. Your medication needs will likely change over time. Because diabetes can be progressive, many people eventually need higher doses, additional medications, or insulin to maintain blood sugars in their target range.

INSULIN TREATMENTS FOR TYPE 1 AND TYPE 2 DIABETES

If even small amounts of carbohydrates are spiking your blood sugars, then it's time to consider insulin. When your doctor prescribes insulin, the process of determining the right dosages may be trial and error. This is especially true if your sleep schedule, meals, and activity levels vary a lot from day to day or if you are under a significant amount of stress.

Basal Insulin

In people with type 1 diabetes, a long-acting basal insulin is the most common treatment. It lasts for about 24 hours and acts evenly during that time. Alternately, you can use an insulin pump to deliver small amounts of rapid-acting insulin (or less commonly, regular insulin) throughout the day.

People with type 2 diabetes who are unable to achieve their target blood sugars with lifestyle changes and multiple non-insulin medications will also benefit from basal insulin. The general strategy is to slowly increase the amount each day until your blood sugars are consistently in the target range when you wake up.

If you need basal insulin and are not taking enough, your blood sugars will be consistently high or hard to control. On the other hand, if you take too much, then you will have frequent low blood sugars. Getting this step right is critical to success.

In most patients, when A1cs are above 7.5% (average blood sugar of 187 mg/dL [10.4 mmol/L]), clinical guidelines recommend taking higher doses of basal insulin. However, identifying confounders may be required.

Bolus Insulin

Most people with type 1 diabetes should be taking rapid-acting insulin at meal times, and to correct high blood sugars. Some people with type 2 diabetes also find they need rapid-acting insulin to be successful.

The Rule of Threes is especially effective at measuring how much insulin you need to cover a meal or to correct a high blood sugar. It takes a lot of practice to figure out how your insulin needs vary throughout the day. Remember to focus on one thing at a time.

The timing of your bolus insulin dose also matters. Many health care providers recommend dosing insulin 15 to 30 minutes before each meal. This lets the insulin

CURB COSTS WITH NPH INSULIN

Unfortunately, long-acting insulins can be expensive, about $200 per vial. To minimize expense, some people must turn to NPH insulin (at $80 to $90 per vial) as basal insulin, even though it only lasts 18 to 22 hours and has a significant peak in action. Its effectiveness also varies based on where it is injected. To smooth out the delivery, NPH insulin is typically injected twice a day, with the morning injection at a higher dose than the shot later in the day to avoid low sugar levels during the night.

DON'T "OVERSHOOT" INSULIN TO LOWER THE HIGHS

When your blood sugar is higher than 180 mg/dL (10 mmol/L), the amount you need to lower it by 10 mg/dL (0.6 mmol/L) will be greater than when you have more normal blood sugars, near 100 mg/dL (5.6 mmol/L). Also, the lower the blood sugar, the faster the fall in blood sugar levels will be with the same amount of insulin. Therefore, it is important to be careful about giving yourself multiple, large doses of insulin even if your blood sugars are 500 mg/dL (27.8 mmol/L) or higher. You don't want to aim to go straight to 100 mg/dL (5.6 mmol/L) because the risk of overshooting and going too low is great.

Let's say you give yourself a hefty, but not too hefty, dose of insulin. It starts to come down, but not fast enough for your liking. So you give yourself another large dose. Because insulin can stay active in the body for more than four hours, these multiple large doses given close together can "stack," leading to severe and unexpected low blood sugars. It is often better to deliver smaller amounts of insulin and give them a chance to start working, even though it feels unpleasant in the meantime.

begin working at about the same time the sugar reaches your blood. This approach can be tricky if you're not in control of the timing of your meals. At a restaurant, for example, if food is served later than expected, your insulin will start working whether you want it to or not and could lead to a significant and embarrassing low sugar. Only employ this approach if you have control over when the food will be served.

Managing Multiple Medications

Sometimes, people with diabetes end up taking too many medications to manage diabetes. If you are taking more than three medications and still not reaching your A1c goals, then something is not working well enough.

Perhaps you've started experiencing a little more back pain or are getting head-aches. This can increase your need for medication or make the medications you are on ineffective. Talk to your doctor about re-evaluating your needs. The solution often requires managing the confounder. In the case of chronic stress or pain, it could require long-acting basal insulin to meet the increased needs of pain management.

Some medications, including antidepressants and steroids, can make diabetes harder to manage. You may want to speak with your doctor or pharmacist to ensure that the non-diabetes medications you are taking don't impact your blood sugars. The key here is not necessarily the amount of medications that you are on, but their effectiveness and the side effects. Listen to your body.

BEWARE A MISDIAGNOSIS OF TYPE 2 DIABETES

If you have been told that you have type 2 diabetes and it seems to be quickly worsening, there is a chance you have been misdiagnosed. This is especially common for people in their 20s and 30s. Someone can develop type 1 diabetes—formerly called "juvenile" diabetes—at any age. Those who develop type 1 diabetes later in life have been frequently misdiagnosed with type 2 diabetes.

If you suspect this is a possibility, request a C-Peptide test, which measures how much insulin your body is producing. If your body produces little-to-no insulin shortly after diagnosis, this is a strong signal that you have type 1 diabetes. Manny Hernandez, founder of the Diabetes Hands Foundation, went through such a misdiagnosis.

NEW MEDS CAN CHANGE INSULIN NEEDS

Some medications may reduce your need for insulin. When adding a new medication to your treatment plan, be aware that it could change the amounts of insulin that you need to take. Ask your doctor about this concern.

Taken by Surprise with Type 1

I was thirty years old when I went to the doctor for my annual checkup. The blood work returned, and my primary care physician told me I had high fasting blood sugars. He said this meant I had diabetes. Over the next six months, we tried five or six variations of metformin. None of them worked. I began to worry that there was a problem.

I had been training for the Valley of the Sun half marathon in Phoenix, and it must have been suppressing my blood sugars, because when I stopped training, it became impossible to keep numbers in my target range. Soon, I couldn't keep them below 150 mg/dL (8.3 mmol/L).

My doctor humbly said, "I don't know what else I can do." He referred me to an endocrinologist, who checked my C-Peptide levels to see how much insulin I was producing. When the results came back, the endocrinologist said my body was producing very little insulin and added, "You have type 1 diabetes."

The fact that it was a chronic condition hit me right then. I've been on insulin for twelve years now.

What Works?

When you try the obvious things to lower blood sugars and they don't work, it's time to refer back to the confounders listed at the start of this chapter. Are you having unrecognized low blood sugars? Are you having frequently interrupted sleep due to undiagnosed sleep apnea? Do you have emotional stress that you're not consciously aware of? Are you in physical pain?

In the absence of confounders, a combination of reducing carbohydrates, increasing physical activity, and taking insulin (or enhancing it with medication) will always lower your blood sugars.

Chapter 5

Step 2: Limit the Lows

If you successfully manage your high blood sugars, you are bound at some point to experience a low blood sugar.

Two of the largest long-term studies of diabetes, DCCT (Diabetes Control and Complications Trial) and ACCORD (Action to Control Cardiovascular Risk in Diabetes), highlighted the challenges of aiming for blood sugars close to the normal range. In each case, those who were achieving among the best results had problems with low blood sugars.

In fact, low blood sugars were so prevalent in the DCCT that it almost ended the study early out of safety concerns,[11] while the ACCORD trial was discontinued because of cardiac-related deaths in the group approaching A1c levels of 6% and lower. Follow-ups to the ACCORD study found that much of the risk was attributed to patients with a higher risk of heart disease, particularly older patients.[28] (For those who are younger and healthier, there is little evidence that aiming for a lower A1c raises your risk of heart attack.)

This is the fundamental balancing act in diabetes. We know that lower sugar levels lead to fewer long-term complications. At the same, they increase your risk for too-low blood sugars.

In the years since these studies, tools available to manage diabetes have improved considerably. There are now more accurate blood glucose meters, better classes of medications, long-acting insulins, and a better understanding of how diabetes actually works. We can reach for lower blood sugar targets with less risk than before. Still, low blood sugars occur too frequently and remain a real problem.

We believe that by using the processes in this book, especially in this chapter, you can achieve your personal goals while minimizing the risks of low blood sugars in ways that would have been impossible twenty years ago.

WHY LOWS MATTER

Low blood sugars are associated with both short- and long-term risks.[29]

In the short-term, low blood sugars don't feel very good. Your skin becomes clammy and sweaty. You feel shaky, anxious, and irritable. Low blood sugar can give you headaches and make it hard to think clearly. As your body becomes desperate for sugar, you may become insatiably hungry. When your brain is starved of sugar, the risk of bad things happening grows enormously. Your judgment can fail. Your reaction time slows. Your ability to respond to or recognize low sugars is damaged. If your blood sugar drops too low, it can lead to seizure, coma, and death.

If you have high blood sugars for an extended period of time, you may experience symptoms of low blood sugar even when you are above the normal range. Your brain has gotten used to the higher levels and senses that something is wrong when it isn't. These symptoms can be especially severe if your sugar levels are dropping rapidly, which can happen when you start on a new medication or insulin. By gradually lowering your blood sugars closer to your target range, these feelings will dissipate in two to three weeks. Your body will adjust so that low sugar symptoms only appear when your sugars approach about 65 mg/dL (3.6 mmol/L) or lower.

Some people have trouble identifying symptoms of low blood sugars until it's too late. This is called hypoglycemia unawareness, and we will talk about how to work through it later in this chapter. First, let's look at how Harry learned to recognize a potentially life-threatening low.

Keep on Truckin'

Low blood sugars were a problem for Harry, who worked for a mid-western trucking company.

Harry had hid his diabetes from his boss so he could continue working as a truck driver. After all, he only took a small dose of insulin at night and a pill in the morning.

On a hot summer day, Harry had unloaded his truck twice and was getting ready to leave when he was assigned an emergency delivery to a factory, two hours away. He would not be home before midnight. He delivered the load to the customer and was on the way back to the truck depot when a thunderstorm opened up. The cab was stifling hot. Harry was sweating and struggled to stay focused on the road.

Harry doesn't remember when the truck left the highway. It slowed after hitting a small tree before tipping on its side and grinding to a stop, fracturing his skull. The paramedics measured his blood sugar at a very low 38 mg/dL (2.1 mmol/L). Fortunately, Harry survived. He was banged up, but the paramedics were able to treat his low blood sugars and stabilize them.

But Harry lost his job and felt ashamed of his mistake.

He went to his doctor for help, afraid that the next time, he might not be so lucky. His doctor referred him to a course called Blood Glucose Awareness Training (BGAT). After successfully completing the course, Harry went to his boss and got his job back, though he had some limitations on how far he could drive.

One day four years later, Harry was filling the gas tank of his car, struggling to figure out how much to pay. The feeling was vaguely familiar to Harry. He remembered the last time he felt this way. It was the last thing he remembered before the truck left the road.

Harry checked his blood sugar. It was 46 mg/dL (2.6 mmol/L). He ate a snack and waited thirty minutes. He still felt uneasy about his ability to drive, but when he checked his blood sugar again, it was up to 160 mg/dL (8.9 mmol/L). Harry had another small snack and drove home.

On the drive home, Harry was thankful for BGAT course he had completed after the truck accident. The program had showed him how to listen when he felt "different." It may have saved his life—and somebody else's.

When Low Sugars Look Like Dementia

Elderly people taking medications for diabetes may appear to be demented and incapable of social interactions or even the activities of daily living. They may in fact have these problems. However, if a loved one taking *any* blood-sugar lowering agent seems to drift into a dementia-like state, examine nighttime sugar levels (or preferably, six days of continuous glucose monitoring) before accepting a diagnosis of dementia. There may be no other sign that low sugars are occurring, and daytime sugars may be in a satisfactory range. Apparent dementia may be nothing other than hypoglycemia, as Lee's story shows.

....

A Sugar Test Changed His Future

Lee had been diagnosed with type 2 diabetes after his 67th birthday, and he was still taking the same medication twelve years later. His annual visits to the doctor revealed no reason to change the medicines, since his A1c was always between 6.5% and 7.0%. In fact, they were better since his wife had died because he was hardly eating the way he did when she was cooking for him. Still, his life had changed dramatically. A CPA for 42 years, he had sold his accounting firm and now was alone.

Lee's niece, Charlotte, came to visit one day and found him uncharacteristically disheveled. He couldn't tie his shoelaces by himself. She took him to the hospital for evaluation, where dementia was diagnosed. She was told it was not likely to be reversible. Charlotte was puzzled because when she last visited her uncle just five weeks before, he was doing okay with activities and planning a trip to visit his son 3,000 miles away. He'd been impeccably dressed and smiling when he greeted her at the door.

Charlotte went to see her endocrinologist, Dr. Ann, about a thyroid problem and asked if she had any insights about her uncle. Dr. Ann asked if he was taking any sugar-lowering pills. Charlotte didn't know, but she knew her uncle did have diabetes. At Charlotte's urging, Dr. Ann agreed to review Lee's situation. When she arrived in the hospital, she found him being wheeled towards the elevator on his way to a nursing home. Dr. Ann insisted he be brought back to his bed for an evaluation. The head nurse objected, but Dr. Ann refused to relent, and it's a good thing. A simple blood sugar check changed his life. Lee had prolonged low blood sugars, not dementia, and after an easy treatment, he left the hospital with Charlotte and drove home himself before he took her out to dinner to celebrate.

WHEN LOWS ARE MOST LIKELY

A variety of things cause low blood sugars, from exercise to drinking alcohol. Let's take a closer look at the main causes.

Increased Activity

Physical activity is very effective at lowering blood sugars. Being more active than usual increases your risk of having low blood sugar. This is especially true if you are doing something that you don't think of as physical activity, like cleaning the house or playing Frisbee on the beach.

If you are taking insulin, increased activity levels can make the insulin work more effectively, dropping your blood sugar faster than expected. This is especially true if you inject insulin into an active limb, like your arm if you're playing tennis or your leg while you're hiking.

CAN LOWS CAUSE IRREVERSIBLE DAMAGE?

A number of studies have examined whether low blood sugars over the long term cause irreversible damage. Many people who have had frequent, severe low blood sugars show no problems decades later. And yet some have gone on to experience debilitating cognitive problems like memory loss or difficulty with calculations. Based on study results, however, it's fair to say that most people experience no long-term complications from low blood sugars.

Taking Too Much Medication or Insulin

When you take something that lowers blood sugars, the dose is usually based on the combination of carbohydrate intake and physical activity. If you eat fewer carbs, your sugar levels may become lower, sooner than you expect.

Matching insulin or medication dosages to carbohydrates presents extra challenges. The more carbohydrates you eat at once, the harder it is to figure out the right dosage. This is a key reason why you should avoiding eating big meals that are very high in carbohydrates.

If your injection is surprisingly painful, you may have injected insulin into a muscle rather than under your skin. There, it acts extremely quickly and can lead to severe, hard-to-correct low blood sugars.

Drinking Alcohol

Adding alcohol to the mix introduces more challenges. Alcohol preoccupies your liver so that it is unable to manufacture and release sugar into your bloodstream to counteract a low blood sugar. This can lead to severe low blood sugars many hours after you stop drinking. Because people often drink in the evenings, this leads to a very dangerous situation while you are sleeping.

Remember that many drinks contain a lot of carbohydrates even though the alcohol itself does not. A rum and regular Coke has up to 40 g of carbohydrates—about as much as a cup of pasta—while a rum and Diet Coke has zero. Beers typically have between 5 g and 15 g of carbohydrates, and wine has about 5 g per glass.

Problems Absorbing Food

A variety of things can change the way your body absorbs food. For example, some medications slow down digestion, leaving unabsorbed food in your stomach. An illness, like the flu or food poisoning, can cause vomiting or diarrhea, another example of unabsorbed food.

Digestive Conditions

Other medical conditions may impact how your body digests carbohydrates. These include celiac disease, which can cause diarrhea, or gastroparesis, which slows down the stomach emptying, delays digestion, and postpones sugar absorption.

Hormonal Irregularities

Hormones in your body impact how much sugar your body creates and releases daily. Adrenal insufficiency and growth hormone insufficiency can increase your sensitivity to insulin. Likewise, problems with your body's processing of glucagon, a hormone that tells your liver to release sugar, can have similar effects. Low thyroid hormone levels don't directly impact how your body releases sugar, but can slow the process. Additionally, low thyroid hormone levels slow digestion and may cause lethargy, which can make it harder for people to recognize low blood sugars. If you have frequent and unexpected low blood sugars, it's worth having your doctor check for these hormonal problems.

LOW SUGARS ON THE GO (CLAIR'S STORY)

When you're busy or preoccupied, it's harder to recognize a low blood sugar. Clair was taken completely by surprise at the Ninth Avenue Diner in Manhattan.

....

Not What She (or the Doctor) Ordered

It was 11:30 on a Saturday morning by the time Clair found a place to eat lunch. She had rushed out of her house to catch the train, fueled by a cup of coffee and an apple.

The Ninth Avenue Diner was on a corner two blocks from the railroad station. Smells of bacon and pastries wafted through the open doors to the street. Clair was drawn in and took a seat at the counter. She studied the menu and picked out roast chicken, peas, and corn.

A gruff counter man approached her. "What would you like, lady?"

"The roast chicken, without the skin, please. I would like the peas and the corn without the butter," Clair responded.

"Drink?" the counter man asked.

"Some tea, please, with a non-sugar sweetener and skim milk."

The man brought a cup of hot water with a teabag, sugar, and cream and quickly disappeared back into the kitchen. Clair grew frustrated. Where was the skim milk and sweetener?

Then she was feeling shaky and not just from annoyance. She could feel her blood sugars dropping. Uncomfortable checking it in front of the other diners, she decided to just wait for her food. (She thought about eating a sugar packet, but that would look silly.)

When her food appeared, the chicken was covered with greasy skin, and the corn, peas, and toast were bathed in a buttery liquid. She dreaded asking the rude server to fix it all.

Then the counterman saw her staring at the food. "Is something wrong?" he grumbled.

"Yes," she said in a louder voice than she intended. "This is not what I ordered!"

"This is chicken, corn, and peas, lady. That is what you ordered! What's the matter with it? I didn't get complaints from anybody else today."

By this time, everyone else in the diner knew Clair was having a problem. She sensed it and looked around her.

"I have diabetes. I have to eat a certain way. I cannot eat this. I asked for no butter on my vegetables and no skin on the chicken, and I don't want butter on my bread!"

The counterman was frustrated. "You came to the wrong place, lady," he said. "We don't serve that kind of stuff here."

One of the other customers laughed and said to her companion, "That's for sure!"

Clair was desperate. "Listen," she said. "My sugar is low. Get me some juice." Then, against her will, she began to weep, embarrassed and shaky.

The counterman's expression softened. "What kind of juice do you want?"

"Any juice. Orange, apple, cranberry, anything!"

Suddenly a large glass of orange juice appeared on the counter. She turned and saw a very concerned gentleman from a nearby table. "I put two packs of sugar in it," he said. "Drink it. It just came to my table, I didn't drink any of it. I know about diabetes. It's okay." He gave her a smile and returned to his table.

Clair drank it. The counter man set another glass down in front of her. "Is that alright? Are you okay, lady?" He asked quietly. "I'll get your food."

A few minutes later, he came back with chicken with no skin and fresh corn and peas with no butter. The bread was lightly toasted and with a small tub of margarine on the side. A waitress was with him and asked if Clair needed anything else.

Clair nodded; she was okay. She wiped the tears from her eyes and face. She ate her meal in silence, paid the bill, thanked the other customer for his kindness, and left the diner feeling thoroughly humiliated.

....

Clair learned a couple of important lessons from her experience.

- She couldn't always feel a low blood sugar coming when she was on the go.
- She had to make sure to always have a source of sugar in her purse.

How to Treat Lows

To treat a low blood sugar, your body needs either sugar or a glucagon injection. We will talk about glucagon in a bit.

Many health care professionals recommend treating a low blood sugar with 15 grams of carbohydrates, waiting 15 minutes to allow your blood sugars to rise, and checking again. If they are not getting close to your target range, repeat the process. It can be very difficult to resist the urge to eat extra carbohydrates. Your body is sending your brain a primal message to consume as many carbohydrates as possible. Resisting the urge is not easy, and sometimes doesn't happen, which can lead to high blood sugars.

The types of carbohydrates you eat make a big a difference. If you need to raise sugar levels quickly, eat simple sugars, avoiding sugar that's mixed with fat or protein unless you have no other options. Chocolate, which is mixed with fat, does a very poor job of raising blood sugars quickly. So does a glass of milk, whether whole or skim.

Dextrose is the best form of sugar to use. You can find it in glucose tablets, many candies (such as Pixy Stix, SweeTARTS, and Sprees), some sugary drinks, and glucose gels. Orange juice, regular soda, and many other drinks contain sugar in other forms such as fructose or glucose. These will work, but not as fast as dextrose. It's wise to stock your pantry, purse, and nightstand with products containing dextrose. Read the ingredients.

If your low blood sugar is caused by long-acting insulin or medication (especially sulfonylureas), you will be at risk of continued low blood sugars. You may have to eat extra carbohydrates until the dose is no longer active in your body. Sulfonylureas can remain active in your body, lowering sugar levels, for five days after you take them. Talk to your doctor, nurse, CDE, or pharmacist, look it up, and make sure you under-stand how each of your blood-sugar lowering medications works.

Glucagon Can Save a Life

If someone is unconscious, the only effective treatments are a glucagon injection or sugar delivered through an IV. Call an ambulance immediately before helping some-one who is unconscious. Do not pour a drink or food into someone's mouth. If they can't swallow it, they may choke and die. If you put your finger in someone's mouth and they have a seizure, their mouth may clamp down and separate your fingers from your hand. This is not a pleasant situation.

Glucagon injections can be challenging to administer if you've never practiced before. Glucagon can't be stored as a liquid without quickly losing effectiveness. To use it, you must mix together two different ingredients, a liquid and a powder, in a syringe to create an injectable glucagon solution.

The good part is that once you have the mixture, it is very easy to deliver. Just give the injection under the skin, in the arms, legs, or into muscle. You can even give it through clothes. It is a forgiving process. This is a lifesaving action, one that prevents a seizure.

After giving a glucagon injection, turn the person on their side in case they vomit and wait for an ambulance or take them immediately to the hospital if that's not an option. The person will usually recover in ten to fifteen minutes and feel groggy, irritable, and sometimes combative. They are waking up from unconsciousness and may not remember or understand what just happened.

REGAIN AWARENESS OF YOUR LOW BLOOD SUGARS

As we said earlier, frequent low blood sugars over time can cause your body to get used to them so much that you'll stop feeling symptoms. This is called hypoglycemia unawareness. Meanwhile, your body's natural protective response to low blood sugars—putting more sugar into your bloodstream—becomes less and less effective. This can lead to prolonged, severe low blood sugars.

It's a dangerous combination: the lows get worse at the same time that you lose the ability to recognize them, and your body becomes less effective in responding.

The good news is that it is possible to regain your awareness of low blood sugars, as Mel did in our introduction when he used a continuous glucose meter to become familiar with his low blood sugars, and then avoid them. The goal is to go for a long period without experiencing any low blood sugars. This can be an unpleasant process. You'll need to pay very close attention to what's happening in your body. And you may need to keep your blood sugars higher than you like.

PRACTICE MAKES GLUCAGON INJECTION PERFECT!

We highly recommend asking your doctor for a glucagon practice kit. Regular glucagon kits also have an expiration date, usually four to six months. If your glucagon has expired, it is an excellent time to grab an orange and practice on it. Be sure to replace expired glucagon—it can save a life!

A standard blood glucose meter is often inadequate for recognizing low blood sugars. We highly recommend using a continuous glucose meter to regain awareness of low sugars. After about three weeks, you should start to be able to feel your low blood sugars again.

Err on the Side of Safety

Low blood sugars are the most immediately dangerous side effect of diabetes. You want to avoid situations like those experienced by Harry the truck driver, Clair at the diner, or Mel as much as possible.

What's the solution? Err on the side of being high, rather than low, when deciding how much insulin or medication to take when eating or mitigating effects of alcohol. When in doubt, take less insulin than you need and more later if you need it. You can always give yourself more insulin, but you can't take it away. If you have recurring low blood sugars, this especially applies to you.

....

Lolita's Awakening

It was late in the evening when I was called to consult on a patient in a suburban hospital. The elderly woman was lying in her bed asleep but askew, her dinner tray untouched on a table too far away to reach from the bed. Her dinner had been served hours before, and she had not eaten, and if she woke up now and wanted to eat, she wouldn't be able to without calling for help.

I called her name, Lolita, and shook her gently. No response. Then I spoke louder, closer to her ear, and she still didn't respond. I immediately called out for a nurse and started going down my mental checklist. There was no evidence of any major illness, but her skin was cold and wet when I touched her arm. Her vital signs were normal.

Looking at her untouched meal, I started to worry. She had been prescribed insulin at each meal to process the carbohydrates she was eating. If she didn't eat those carbohydrates, the insulin she received would push her blood sugar to dangerously low levels, creating her coma-like state. I directed the nurse to immediately add sugar to her IV.

Within moments, Lolita's eyes flickered open. She became alert enough to look right at me and ask, "Who are you and why are you here in my room?"

She then asked for her daughter. The nurse informed us that her daughter, Leona, was coming. When I asked the patient what her name was, she curtly replied, "Ask my daughter."

Lolita was 84 years old. After sixteen years with diabetes, she had become progressively more forgetful and had a long history of high sugar levels "all the time." Now, she was prone to falling asleep in a room full of people. The family was familiar with the coldness of her skin and her sweating.

They thought it was because her blood sugars were always so high. They had increased her medication dosage multiple times in recent weeks, in consultation with her doctor.

When I arrived in her room to find her unconscious, her blood sugar was a very low 38 mg/dL (2.1 mmol/L). Before leaving to see another patient, I adjusted Lolita's medication.

On my rounds the next evening, I found Lolita and her daughter, Leona, waiting for me. Lolita was awake and alert but still deferred all questions to her daughter. Leona had tears streaming down her face. "What do I do? How do I deal with this? Who will take care of her if it isn't me?"

Leona was facing a common concern: being forced to move a parent to a nursing home for round-the-clock care. But that's not how this success story ended.

Three days later, Lolita went home to live with Leona and Leona's husband. Within three weeks, there were no more low blood sugars and less frequent high blood sugars, and then only when Lolita found the cookies in the pantry. During the next four years, Lolita took the steps outlined in this book and was never hospitalized for her diabetes again.

Lolita and Leona's Action Plan

To eliminate Lolita's low sugars, we made sure she ate all her meals when presented. If she ate less, she would take less medication. In this way, her serious low sugar episodes disappeared, along with the afternoon sleepiness she had experienced for several years. Within three days, her sugars stabilized and began to improve.

Leona worked with her health care team to understand and proactively manage her mother's diabetes. At first, she was worried that she would do the wrong thing, but we reassured her by reminding her how much better her mother looked now than during those days in the hospital. Lolita liked all the attention she was getting and was grateful to have more energy.

Months later, during one of their routine doctor visits, Leona and the doctor spent the whole time talking about Lolita and the things they were doing to manage her diabetes. As the visit ended, her doctor turned to Lolita and asked. "What do you think about how Leona is helping you with your diabetes?"

In a very matter-of-fact tone, she smiled and said, "I don't hate my diabetes anymore. Without it, I never would have gotten to spend so much time with my daughter." Their smiles filled the room. Lolita's last years were lived in the comfort that only a caring family can provide, instead of a nursing home facility that would have spent the money she had saved for her grandchildren's college tuition.

Lolita's and Leona's experiences are typical among people who follow the *Thriving with Diabetes* plan outlined in these pages. By checking blood sugars strategically and making small changes, they came to understand why the sugars changed. Leona got out in front of her mother's diabetes problems before unwanted things happened and enjoyed life in spite of the challenges that diabetes presents.

SUPPORT FOR CONTINUOUS MONITORING

When you talk to your doctor about getting a continuous glucose monitor or sensor to fix low blood sugar unawareness, ask for a referral to an endocrinologist for more intensive support. It can take months to be able to fully recognize your symptoms again. Once you have had hypoglycemia unawareness, you are at risk of it happening again. You'll feel good about taking early action to prevent it.

Chapter 6

Step 3: Use Your Best to Fix the Rest

One big challenge with diabetes is its complexity. You are taking over the management of a system with more than a hundred moving pieces. It's understandably hard. This chapter is where the magic begins. We will show you how to make diabetes simpler. But how do you take a system with so many parts and make it more predictable? Easier to manage?

We believe most people approach diabetes backwards. They start by looking at the highest numbers. They start by looking at the past. This makes sense on one level. You want to fix the high blood sugars because they cause the long-term complications of diabetes. That is a good gut instinct. But the high blood sugars, so long as they are not leading to diabetic ketoacidosis or other immediate problems, are probably not urgent. You want to fix them, but they are not going to cause a problem over the next few days. Long-term complications take years to develop.

It makes sense that by looking at the past, we might predict what will make blood sugars go up and down. Diabetes, though it may not seem like it at times, is predictable. If we had enough knowledge about the past, we could use it to influence the future. The problem is that we very rarely collect the kind of information we need to understand what has already happened.

The secret to success is a strategy we call "Use Your Best to Fix the Rest." Rather than starting with what's broken, start with what's working and move forward. Begin by noting a good blood sugar level, see where it goes awry, and figure out what happened to cause the change. When you understand when and why things have gone off track, you'll have an opportunity to fix them *before* they rise or fall.

This chapter is about knowing what to collect, when to collect it, and what to do with the information. Instead of looking backwards, we will show you how to look forward.

Looking In-Range Gains Traction

The ability to chart blood sugars in real-time has helped us understand that diabetes is not just about lowering high blood sugars, but understanding how our daily activities cause our blood sugars to go up and down. The idea of focusing on keeping blood sugars in-range is a newer concept. It's only been in the last twenty years, and especially the last ten with the availability of continuous glucose meters, that this has been the goal. For some people who have had diabetes for a long time, the changes in management philosophy can be hard to process.

Let's look at the experience of Mary Ellen, a 94-year-old woman who had been living with type 1 diabetes for more than 70 years.

Bittersweet Advances

Mary Ellen recalled the glass syringes that she had boiled in water and the huge needles she had sharpened on a stone as a teenager. She would visit the hospital so her doctor could check her sugars. He would take some urine, mix it in a test tube, and measure the change in colors. She knew when they were high by how frequently she had to urinate.

Mary Ellen's life was miraculously transformed when home testing of urine became available. Suddenly, she could take a strip into her bathroom and know immediately how high her sugars were. This felt like a "real-time" reading to Mary Ellen. But it was not. Measuring sugar in urine gives you a rough estimate of what your blood sugars were many hours before, and it's an incomplete picture. There is no concept of looking at low blood sugars. You can only measure high blood sugars, let alone normal or low ones.

For Mary Ellen, diabetes had been purely a matter of lowering high blood sugars. With limited information, she had less time to react to high blood sugars. This put her at a far higher risk of diabetic ketoacidosis than people experience today—and DKA was a far more lethal condition than it is today.

In the 1980s, meters for checking blood sugars at home became widely available. This was an improvement over checking sugar in urine, but still not very accurate. Yet each year, the accuracy and reliability for measuring high blood sugars improved. By the late 1980s and early 1990s, doctors began looking not just at the highs, but the lows. They studied how they were connected and later began looking at the rhythms of diabetes in earnest.

Mary Ellen had never thought much about low sugars, and she didn't believe it was possible to maintain sugars in a "normal range." This was not part of her thinking when she developed diabetes, nor did she think it was possible fifty years afterward. When urged to look less at the highs and more at the big picture of her body's rhythms, she bristled.

She only wanted to prick her finger when she was urinating too much. But, to her credit, Mary Ellen gave it a go. When using a meter, it was hard for her to believe she was getting a number. A real number! Urine testing never did that. It had always been "way too much," "too much," or "less than too much." In the past, she would take insulin and wait until the next day to see how well it worked. With her blood glucose meter, as she came to trust it, she liked seeing how she was doing in hours instead of days.

But here was a new worry for Mary Ellen. Sometimes, her insulin would push her sugar levels too low. In the past, she would feel hungry and eat. Now, she was getting low numbers, and they scared her. When it was too low, she got the shaky fear that she might die at any moment. (She learned that this wasn't true). She learned to eat some glucose and wait 15 minutes and test again. The fear lessened, but didn't go away.

All this extra information about her highs and lows made it appear like her diabetes was moving much faster and was much more complex. After living with the condition for over 70 years, none of this was easy to accept. Diabetes used to be so much simpler.

We know far more about diabetes now than ever. We've gone from not nearly enough information to the fear of information overload. Yet, these news tools have enabled previously impossible levels of health, wellbeing, and long-term success.

HOW TO USE YOUR BEST TO FIX THE REST

Instead of looking for sugars that are too high or too low, look for parts of your day where sugar levels are where you want them to be. Is it first thing in the morning on workdays? In the late afternoon, before dinner? The secret is to find a part of the week where your blood sugars are consistently pretty good and you feel comfortable about them.

Most people have periods where their diabetes is predictable. This tends to happen when you do the same things at the same time of day. If you sleep at the same time and wake up at the same time, your sugar trends during that period will tend to be similar.

If you wake up in the middle of night or have stress-fueled nightmares, this can change. Eating a very late dinner, drinking alcohol, taking different doses of medication, or anticipating a stressful next day can also change your sugar trends. If you are on such a blood sugar roller coaster, diabetes becomes less predictable. This is especially the case if you are taking too much medication and experiencing lots of low blood sugars or if you have one of the major "confounders" we discuss below.

There are two general strategies for increasing predictability that tend to work well for people. The first is to start early in the day and extend the periods that work. Successes in the morning help resolve afternoon problems without you having to do anything else. The second strategy is to focus on your multipliers.

The Power of Multipliers

Multipliers are the activities that you do most frequently. If you can find a successful way to manage your sugars during that activity, you can multiply your success by repeating the behavior. For example, most of us eat the same breakfast on most mornings. It might be scrambled eggs and a piece of toast. Figure out how to manage your blood sugars during that breakfast. Do you eat it five times a week? You just multiplied that success times five!

For something to be a true multiplier, three things must be true:

1. The event must be the same. . .
You're eating the same food, performing the same exercise routine, or doing the same housework.

2. . . .at the same time of day.
Remember, your body's hormonal rhythms change throughout the day. A meal eaten first thing in the morning may have a different impact on your blood sugars than if it is eaten later in the day. (For those taking insulin, your doctor may be prescribing a different "insulin-to-carbohydrate ratio" at different times of day to account for this.)

3. You have accounted for overlapping activities.
A lousy night's sleep may cause your breakfast blood sugars to be different in the morning. An unusually busy day of walking around the home, school, or workplace will change how dinner affects your blood sugars.

We'll tease apart the causes and effects between multiple activities further on. For now, to check how predictable they are, we use the Rule of Threes discussed in Chapter 5.

1. Check your blood sugar.
2. Do something.
3. Check your blood sugar again.

If you repeat this at the same time on three different days and get the same results, you'll know that the impact on your blood sugars is predictable. Predictability is part of the magic.

BE WARY OF CONFOUNDERS

As you look for patterns, be aware that a number of things can completely disrupt your blood sugars. We call them "confounders" because they cause confusion. These are game stoppers. They can disrupt your diabetes for weeks at a time. If you keep finding yourself in confusing situations, stop and look for confounders from the list below. They can throw a wrench into the gears of a perfectly predictable period:

- **Medication snafus**
  - *Mixing up medications.* If you mistakenly switch doses of medications, it can cause major issues. This is especially true if you take a rapid-acting insulin in place of a long-acting one. It will drop your blood sugars like a rock. Be especially careful to avoid mix-ups if you take a long-acting dose of insulin at night.

  - *Doubling up on your pills.* Did you forget if you took your diabetes pills before breakfast today? Be careful about doubling up and putting yourself at risk of a whole day of low blood sugars.

  - *Missing doses or changing the timing.* Some medications are highly sensitive to dose and timing. Be especially careful when your doctor prescribes a new medication or dosing procedure. Drugs taken early in the day can have an unexpected impact later on. If you take multiple medications, they all have different periods when they are working the hardest. Talk to your doctor about when your medications start working, peak, and stop working.

  - *Bad insulin.* Insulin can go bad if it freezes, gets too hot, or too cold. Read the label on your insulin to see how long it keeps after opening and what temperature it needs to be stored at. Insulin doesn't immediately go bad, but gets increasingly less effective over time. If your insulin just doesn't seem to be working well anymore, you may be right.

- **Low blood sugars.** As we discussed earlier, low blood sugars cause a series of changes in your body that can make diabetes unpredictable. Unrecognized low blood sugars can be a major confounder. One side effect of low blood sugars is high blood sugars later. If you only notice the highs, there is a tendency to take too much medication.

- **Bad night's sleep.** Sleep influences your body's rhythm, changing how sensitive you'll be to insulin throughout the day. When your sleep is shortened, interrupted, or skipped, it can cause significant changes in your blood sugars for the entire next day. When traveling across time zones, this can become a major issue. Speak with your doctor about how to adjust your medication dosages and timing while traveling.

- **Stress.** Stress increases your resistance to insulin and leads to high blood sugars. Stress can be caused by physical or emotional pain, temporary illness, or chronic illness. Mild but chronic pain is an often-discounted cause of high blood sugars. If you are starting a new treatment for chronic pain, watch out for low blood sugars.

- **Inaccurate blood sugar tests.** When your blood glucose meter and test strips are not giving accurate results, it's hard to know what to do. Or, if you're not able to wash your hands before checks, you may end up checking things other than the sugar in your blood. Test strips that haven't been stored well can go bad. In rarer cases, the meter can fail. If your results don't make sense, first wash your hands and then check your results against another meter to make sure there's no problem with your testing tools.

- **Failing diabetes devices.** Insulin pumps and continuous glucose meters have components that can fail. Problems with an infusion site for an insulin pump, for example, can lead to prolonged and unexplained high blood sugars. These can be hard to detect quickly.

- **Menstrual cycle or pregnancy.** A woman's menstrual cycle or pregnancy can cause major changes in her body's hormonal rhythms. Women experience different changes during their menstrual cycles, but they tend to be consistent within the individual. Look for patterns in high blood sugars or low blood sugars throughout the different stages of your cycle. The changes may come a few days before or after your period.

- **Other medications like steroids or anti-depressants.** Some medications can cause major changes in your blood sugars. Check with your pharmacist whenever you are prescribed a drug to make sure it does not raise or lower your blood sugars unexpectedly.

We don't want to scare or discourage you. Once you are aware of them, many confounders are easy to recognize. Over time, you will learn to quickly go through your mental checklist, identify the issue, and know what steps to take.

The Role of Physical Pain

As Nancy discovered, being in physical pain can be a strong, unrecognized confounder. Healing her pain reduced her need for insulin.

....

Arthritis & Diabetes—Who Knew?

When Nancy was a girl on the farm, she fell off a horse and dislocated her shoulder. Fifty years later, arthritis was developing in her shoulder and the pain was growing. Her doctor tried a long stream of treatments, painkillers, and anti-inflammatory drugs. She received an injection of steroids, which didn't help but caused her blood sugars to go through the roof.

Finally, her doctor prescribed morphine. Within hours, her blood sugars dropped to within the normal range. She only needed a third of the insulin she had been taking. When she stopped taking the morphine, her insulin needs tripled.

Soon afterward, she had shoulder surgery. As she healed, she no longer needed the large doses of insulin. The surgery fixed her pain, and to her surprise, she quickly lost 40 pounds (18 kg), returning to a weight she hadn't seen since her thirties.

Emotional Triggers

All sorts of strong emotions can disrupt your blood sugars. Fear and guilt are especially powerful, as Jake's story reveals.

Hiding the Truth

Dr. Lewis puzzled over Jake. His blood sugars were consistently high and unresponsive to every medication that she tried, including insulin. When his insulin requirements continued to rise, she admitted him to the hospital for further tests, but found nothing wrong.

Dr. Lewis interviewed Jake about his life, searching for some symptom or stress that could explain his high sugar reactions. He swore up and down there was nothing going on in his personal life or professional life as an accountant. He felt fine.

After a week, she discharged him. There was simply nothing there to fix. Dr. Lewis fell asleep that night frustrated. She so rarely failed to identify what was wrong.

Later that month, the answer came on the front page of the newspaper: "Jake Starling Arrested On Suspicion of Embezzlement."

"So it was stress!" thought Dr. Lewis.

Unseen Triggers

Sometimes, the confounder is something you hide even from yourself.

....

Submerged Grief

William's family and friends marveled at how he handled the tragedy. He had been so close with his mother and handled the funeral arrangements with such thoughtfulness. When he eulogized her, the room careened from tears at his loss to laughter and the good times he remembered. She had breathed joy into all those around her.

Everyone was further surprised when he returned to work a few days later without missing a beat. A few weeks later, he went to his doctor for a routine appointment. His doctor looked over his blood sugars and saw that they were higher than they had been in years, and his A1c had risen a full point.

His doctor advised William to take some time off from his flourishing business to grieve his mother's death. William declined. He promised to contact the doctor if there were any problems. A month later, William was about to begin a business meeting when he sat down at the head of the table and begin to weep uncontrollably.

He left the meeting and went to his doctor's office. His doctor advised him again to take some personal time out of town to experience his grief. At least a week, he said.

William left the next day. When he returned to the doctor ten days later, William felt sad but relieved. His blood sugars were settling back down to prior levels.

....

Disrupted Rhythms

Sometimes, the confounder disrupts your body's rhythms. This is especially common among people who work shifts at different times, like Leah, a nurse.

Perchance to Dream

Leah's sister had died of type 1 diabetes after a second attempted pancreatic transplant a few years ago. Leah knew her diabetes was less of a problem than her sister's had been, but as she was growing older, it was becoming more challenging to manage.

Now things had gotten dramatically more difficult. The hospital where Leah worked had introduced a new shift schedule, throwing everything out of whack. Even worse, she had begun to feel tingling in her fingers and toes. As a nurse, she immediately recognized the symptoms of neuropathy and called her doctor in a panic. Her doctor prescribed a higher insulin dose to bring her sugars down, to no avail. Leah's sugar levels stayed stubbornly high.

Leah's doctor asked her to keep a log of when she was sleeping and the major events in each day. When she brought it back a month later, the doctor quickly noticed that her shifts had been changing, eight hours at a time. She was experiencing the equivalent of jet lag, making her extremely resistant to insulin.

Leah's doctor contacted Leah's hospital, explained the situation to her supervisor, and worked with her to create a schedule that altered Leah's sleep schedule no more than a few hours between days. It worked. Her sugars came down, and her early symptoms of neuropathy went away.

Babies in the House

Some confounders come in tiny, loveable packages.

....

Nourish Yourself First

Georgette was a happy mom. Her son, Jonathan, fell asleep every night at eight o'clock. He woke up hungry every few hours, and she treasured the time she spent snuggling with him in her rocking chair. She had been very worried about how her sugar management would handle frequent wake-ups and breastfeeding, but it was going unexpectedly well.

During the first three months, Jonathan gained eight pounds (3.6 kg). Georgette began to notice that after breast-feeding, she felt ill. One day, when checking her blood sugar before and after breastfeeding, she was surprised to discover her blood sugar had dropped 40 points (2.2 mmol/L), to 50 mg/dL (2.8 mmol/L), in forty minutes.

Georgette put some snacks next to her rocking chair as a reminder to eat before her baby did. It worked, and her blood sugars stopped dropping without making any changes to her medication.

....

HOW TO MANAGE CONFOUNDERS

As we have shown, confounders come in all forms. Identifying them is a critical skill for achieving success. Once you have identified a cofounder, you have three options:

1. **Remove the confounder.** This may mean inviting your mother-in-law to reconsider her housing. (Although asking her to leave might cause stress of a different kind!) Or, a simpler example could be planning your evenings so you can get more consistent sleep.

2. **Fix the confounder.** Say your company takes inventory on Friday, and you spend the day walking around rather than sitting at a desk. You notice this extra activity tends to cause low blood sugars on Friday evenings. You might talk to your doctor about decreasing your diabetes medication or eating an extra snack to fix this issue. Problem solved.

3. **If it's not something you can easily change or fix, account for it.** You recognize that a stressful period has increased your blood sugars, and you probably need to add medication or increase your activity level to manage it. Or, you may decide it's not permanent and ride it out for a few days.

Remember, Keep Track of What Counts

No one likes busywork, so it's good to pay attention to the information you collect. If you are using it to make changes and improve your health, that's a good thing. If you're not using it for anything, it's a waste of your time. If your doctor asks you to check sugar levels at certain times, make sure you understand why and what he or she will do with the information.

Some people with type 2 diabetes are told to check their blood sugar every morning when they wake up. Three months later, they have 90 readings showing pretty much the same blood sugars in the target range. Could they have figured that out in the first week and then just spot-checked a few times a month to make sure it was still true?

This is one of the big reasons why insurance companies have fought against paying for test strips. They are loathe to pay for collection of information that is rarely used to change health outcomes. Too few people are using blood sugar checks to make the types of changes we discuss in this book.

If you are asked to check once a day, consider rotating when you check, to see not just your waking sugar levels, but also your sugars after each of your major meals. Check before and after an event that's likely to change your sugar levels. Having one reading without the other doesn't tell you as much, does it? Diabetes is enough work without collecting unnecessary information.

SPLIT YOUR DAY INTO SEGMENTS

Going back to the idea that your body's rhythms change throughout the day, it makes sense to look at different parts of the day separately. Diving deeply into your whole day is a recipe for burnout. Your patterns are dictated by when you go to sleep, when you wake up, and when you have your meals.

As you Use Your Best to Fix the Rest, start by looking for the time period when your blood sugars are most consistently in your target range. For example, many people wake up with blood sugars in their target range. It's better to look at that one time period for a few days to verify a pattern before looking at another time period.

Identify the Parts Working Well

It's easy to get a quick snapshot of how you are doing with your overall diabetes management. First, you wake up and check your blood sugar. Then you check again before lunch. If you wake up in your target range and are in the target range before lunch and feeling well, then whatever you are doing in between is more or less working.

You can now move on and check your sugar before dinner. If your blood sugars generally stay in the target range from before lunch to before dinner, the afternoons are working too. If you check before bed and you continue to be in the target range, then your whole day is good. If this is the case and your A1c is at target, then you are right where you need to be and no major changes may be necessary.

Now let's look more deeply at each part of the day to understand common issues with meals, physical activity, and the confounders we discussed previously.

When to Check Your Blood Sugar

With meals, you want to check your blood sugar immediately before eating and one hour after the meal. Blood sugars tend to be highest after a meal, so there you will find your peak. Many physicians and nurses recommend checking two or three hours after a meal. This lets you see how well your body was able to handle the meal and get back into the target range.

The challenge with waiting too long after eating to check is that another event, such as physical activity or stress, can impact your blood sugars in the meantime. This makes it harder to understand the causes and effects.

Begin at Night

We begin during the night because your body's rhythms are set by when you go to sleep and when you wake up. Getting a full night of uninterrupted sleep is one of the best things you can do to make your diabetes more predictable.

It's easy to figure out what's happening at night. Check your blood sugar level when you go to bed, in the middle of the night, and right after waking. Yes, this does require waking up in the middle of the night, but not every night. You just need to do it two or three times to confirm what typically happens. You may identify with one of a few common patterns:

Relative Consistency

Your sugars are relatively consistent, modestly rising or falling, with a possible extra rise in the morning as your body prepares to wake up. This is typical; nothing unusual is happening. If this is you, then your blood sugar level should be more predictable in the morning.

Level Falls Too Low

The second pattern is falling asleep, the level falling overnight, and ending up with low blood sugar in the morning. In this case, the low blood sugar will make you more sensitive to insulin in the morning and put you at increased risk for reoccuring low blood sugars all day. There may sometimes be high values between the lows.

A variation is falling asleep in the target range, dropping low, and then having your body recover on its own. This is easy to miss. You fell asleep with a normal blood sugar and woke up higher. Who would suspect a low blood sugar during that time? Yet, there are a number of signs that this is happening. You may wake up with a headache or feeling tired, sick, or groggy. You may have nightmares. You may notice increased sensitivity to medication or insulin and have more low blood sugars in the first half of the day. Check your urine for ketones, as we discussed in Chapter 3.

SCARY UNSEEN LOWS AT NIGHT

There are a variety of confounders to watch out for during the nighttime period: low blood sugars, evening meals, alcohol, medications, and activities. If you tend to eat or be active near bedtime, it can have a major impact on what happens while you sleep.

Please be extra careful to rule out nighttime low blood sugars. Even if you have type 2 diabetes and are unconcerned, this is an important step. Low blood sugars during sleep are one of the most common and unrecognized causes of hard-to-control diabetes of any type.

Low blood sugars are especially common at night. To complicate matters, this is the time when you are asleep and unable to respond, so the lows tend to be prolonged and taxing on your body. To fix nighttime low blood sugars, talk to your doctor about adjusting your medications, activities, or evening snacks.

Asleep and Sugars Up

The third pattern is falling asleep in the target range and your sugars rising overnight. This can be a sign that you are eating too many carbohydrates before bed or not taking enough blood sugar-lowering medication.

The Dawn Phenomenon

Many people wake up with elevated blood sugars in the morning due to the dawn phenomenon. Your body is providing you with extra fuel (i.e., sugar) to get the day started. Some people worry unnecessarily about this typically small increase in levels.

High blood sugars in the morning can also be caused by not taking enough insulin or blood sugar-lowering medications for the food that was eaten the previous evening.

You can determine whether you are experiencing the dawn phenomenon or high blood sugars by checking in the middle of the night. If your blood sugars are normal then and rising later, it's the dawn phenomenon. Otherwise, it's important to look at what was happening before you went to sleep. A 3 a.m. blood sugar check may help to clarify whether you are having a rebound elevation after a low sugar.

Is the morning increase something you really need to worry about? For many people, the dawn phenomenon is a lower rise than they would get after a typical meal. It also tends to extend from an hour or two before waking to a few hours afterwards. If it's a modest and temporary rise, it may not have a significant impact on your overall health and may be safely ignored. Talk to your doctor about whether this is the case for you.

The dawn phenomenon will influence how you manage your morning meal and activities. If you take mealtime medication or insulin, you will likely require more in the morning because you need to manage not just the meal itself, but also the sugar from the dawn phenomenon.

An hour after your morning meal, your blood sugars will be at their peak. You can talk to your doctor about what the appropriate blood sugar level is for you during this time. For most people, medical recommendations say that an increase of around 80 mg/dL (4.4 mmol/L) is acceptable.

As a result of the dawn phenomenon, morning physical activity will also lower blood sugars less than performing the same exercise later in the day. If you do the same exercise at the same time in the morning on three different days, the change in blood sugars should be consistent (absent confounders).

Lunch to Evening

You have successfully made it to lunchtime within your target range. Congratulations!

Once your day gets going, different challenges emerge. You eat more varied meals, do various activities, or experience unexpected stresses. Figuring out how all these confounders influence your blood sugars can be tough. Sometimes, you eat at home; sometimes you eat out. Sometimes, you have the same lunch day after day, or you go out with friends and absent-mindedly eat bread while chatting. The more carbohydrates you eat, the more challenging it becomes to deal with sugar spikes.

Likewise, your activity levels range from planned activities, like a workout, to unplanned treks around a workplace. It makes sense that more complex and varied meals, combined with unpredictable activity levels, make diabetes more challenging to manage during the afternoon.

AFTERNOON LOWS

The symptoms of low blood sugar may feel different in the middle of the day than they do in the morning. People often feel sleepy or unmotivated and don't recognize it because they are involved in activities. Take note of the symptoms of low blood sugars that you experience during this time period and keep an eye out for them in the future. Periodically measure your blood sugars in the mid-afternoon to ensure that you are not having unrecognized lows. It took Lisa almost a decade to make the connection.

Fuzzy Thinking

Lisa had been going to her doctor for many years to improve her diabetes. She was a receptionist in a different doctor's office, getting tired of the long days at work. Every afternoon around 2:00 p.m., she would feel cranky, tired, and fed up with her co-workers.

She felt guilty about all the mistakes she would make.

She never thought to tell her diabetes doctor about it. During one of her check-ups, she mentioned numbness in her hand during the afternoon. Her doctor was concerned about this and her higher than normal A1c. He began to suspect she was experiencing unrecognized low blood sugars followed by high blood sugars.

He asked her if she checked her blood sugar when her hand felt numb.

"No," she confessed sheepishly.

Her doctor advised her to take less insulin at lunchtime and check her blood sugar at the same time for the next few days.

Lisa returned, beaming. Her afternoon grumpiness had been replaced by a surprising burst of extra energy. She thanked the doctor and chastised herself for waiting almost a decade to bring it up.

Getting Ready for Bed

As the day winds down, your main objective is minimizing high blood sugars while avoiding nighttime lows. If your activity levels are greater than usual during the day, you need to be particularly careful about not taking too much medication close to bedtime or propping your blood sugars up with a snack. This is especially important when you're more active than usual. Even casual walking around the mall during the afternoon increases how much sugar your muscles use.

If there is any question about how much medication to take, especially if you experience or suspect low blood sugars at night, talk to your doctor about how to adjust your dosages.

DIFFERENT DAYS, DIFFERENT PATTERNS (JACK'S STORY)

Jack, a junior at State University, was dealing with different schedules on different days, making his diabetes harder to predict.

Unpredictable Afternoons

Jack had two jobs: complete his degree as a mechanical engineer while earning the money to pay for it. On Tuesdays and Thursday, he was in class from 8:00 a.m. to 11:00 a.m. In the afternoons, he would sit, study, and stress. Occasionally, he would over-caffeinate himself. But that's okay, Jack's blood sugars were where he wanted them to be on school days.

On Monday, Wednesdays, and Fridays, he worked 9-to-5 at his internship, assisting a team of mechanical engineers in the design of factory machinery. In the afternoons, he would support a team of repair specialists as they traversed a factory as big as a football field.

On those days, he was waking up where he wanted to be. And his mornings spent sitting and drafting mechanical drawings were predictable. By lunch, he would still be coasting along in a good place. But the afternoons were a different story. Some days he was crashing low at 4:00 p.m., and on others, he was heading to dinner with a blood sugar above 300 mg/dL (16.7 mmol/L).

After a long talk with his doctor, Jack decided to focus on his workday afternoons. This was when his diabetes consistently dropped like a cliff. He started looking at things that varied from day to day. He boiled it down to two key considerations. The first was his lunch. On some days, he brought a brown bag lunch. On others, he went out to a local restaurant and splurged. The second factor was how physically active he was. On some days, he stood next to a machine and tinkered for three hours. On others, he practically jogged from one side of the factory to the other. He never knew what kind of afternoon he was going to have.

Using the Rule of Threes, Jack began checking his levels before lunch and one hour after to see how he was handling his brown bag lunches. That part of his day was fine.

When he went out to lunch, things got dicey. Some days he was up over 300 mg/dL (16.7 mmol/L), but other days he was barely above 180 mg/dL (10 mmol/L). He started carefully logging exactly what he was eating and realized over the following few weeks that the culprit was the appetizers, especially the mozzarella sticks with tomato sauce, which had more carbs than he expected. He also tended to eat more than he planned on eating when he was hungry.

As he thought about it, Jack realized he already knew the problem with his after lunch blood sugars. He had varying levels of physical activity and stress. He could never guess in advance what type of afternoon it was going to be.

He did two things. He started paying close attention to where he was an hour after lunch when he went out with the guys. If his sugars were high, he would worry less about lows in the afternoon. But if he were closer to his target range, he would pay careful attention to how active he was. He also set an alarm on his phone for 3:30 p.m. every afternoon. Sometimes, he would get so busy that he'd forget to check. This was especially true on the days he was most active and likely to have low blood sugar.

Jack also shared with his mentor on the factory floor that he had diabetes. He explained some of the symptoms and showed him how to use a glucagon pen if ever there was a major problem. It turned out that his mentor was better at noticing when he was low in the afternoons than he was.

....

Fix Confounders First

The Use Your Best to Fix the Rest approach works for many, but not all. Diabetes can be complex and hard to understand. Your daily schedule can be chaotic, and you wake up at different times. You could be overwhelmed with stress if a loved one is diagnosed with a heartbreaking illness. You might be diagnosed with arthritis and need to reconsider the patterns that you've come to rely on over the last few years.

When chaos unfolds, your immediate goals change. If things are generally working well, focus on the details. How do you manage weekday lunches? How do you manage exercise? But when things become chaotic, it is time to zoom out and look at the big picture.

Your goal is to get off the blood sugar roller coaster. If your A1c has risen to 10% because your house burned down and you are living out of an apartment, scrambling to rebuild your life, your goal is not perfection. Your goal is to reduce your blood sugar swings until your diabetes is more predictable. This may mean aiming for an A1c of 7.5% instead of 6.5% for a little bit. That's okay. Step back and solve the confounders first. Once your diabetes becomes more predictable, you can Use Your Best to Fix the Rest.

Chapter 7

Step 4: Play with Your Diabetes

S o far, we have focused on the predictable parts of your life. Now it's time to look at how to handle life's little surprises and big changes. We might consider how children cope with the unknown—through constant trial and error, understanding that too big a leap can hurt. To learn the skills you need to thrive, especially in times of upheaval, you need to harness your child-like ability to learn and adapt.

Children are lucky. The world is new and ready to be explored; their sense of safety taking them only as far out on a limb as they can go. As adults, we have the baggage of "dos" and "don'ts" that we've picked up over the years from medical professionals, friends, and headlines. We get fixated on rules we've internalized and forget how to adapt and change. Children have a much more intuitive sense of how the world works. Kids in nurturing environments grow up into capable adults with a wide range of adaptable skills.

Sarah learned a lot by playing with her diabetes. And the skills helped with more than pizza. She came to understand how to handle all sorts of foods.

The Pizza Challenge

Before her diabetes diagnosis, Sarah's favorite meal was pizza at Valentino's. Afterward, she quickly learned it was basically impossible to eat more than a slice without sending her blood sugars on a roller coaster.

Pizza is one of the more challenging foods to eat for diabetes. You start with a lot of dough full of carbohydrates and top it with tomato sauce, which is also full of carbohydrates. Then you add a delicious layer of fatty cheese, which slows down the digestion of all of those carbs. Consider that mealtime insulin lasts about four hours, but pizza can take far longer than that to fully digest.

When Sarah was feeling pretty good about her diabetes management, she swore to herself and her friends that she would master the art of eating three slices of Valentino's pizza.

Her plan was to check her blood sugar before she ate and every two hours until she got back to where she wanted to be.

The first day was a disaster. She had counted 108 grams of carbs, dialed up 7 units of her insulin pen, and endured a devastating low forty minutes later before skyrocketing hours after that. The second attempt wasn't much better. She took less insulin, but still had a severe low and a spike later. Frustrated, she decided to take her insulin later. The third time, 20 minutes after she started eating, she took only six units of insulin.

This worked beautifully: she found her blood sugars were high but not wildly so after two and three hours. The next morning, however, Sarah woke up with blood sugars over 400 mg/dL (22.2 mmol/L). She felt lousy and cursed Valentino's. Thinking back, she realized that her insulin was only lasting four hours and the pizza must have been hanging around in her digestive tract longer than that. She needed her insulin to last longer.

On the fourth attempt, she split the insulin into two doses. She took the first, larger dose about 15 minutes after she started eating and the rest about two hours later when she was getting ready to leave the restaurant. And it worked!

Over the years that followed, Sarah continued to modify and perfect her insulin dosing strategy. She never got it working 100%, but it was good enough that she could enjoy the occasional pizza without dealing with too many consequences the next day. For a slice of Valentino's? It was worth it.

FIRST, ENSURE SAFETY

Let's return to a child climbing a tree. She has a simple sense of safety, climbing until her fear overwhelms her sense of adventure, trying not to get scratched along the way. She stands there, happy and content. Safety for an adult is more expansive. You have a deeper sense of the immediate risks, such as low blood sugars. You may have a long-term fear of losing your health, experiencing pain, and dying early. It is important to both be safe and to feel safe.

You must err on the side of safety when making decisions. This means aiming a little higher if you may go too low or aiming a little lower if you may go too high. It's better to do things in small steps when you are unsure, rather than overshooting your mark. You can always take more medication or eat more carbs, but you can't uninject insulin or remove food from your digestive tract.

To feel safe, you must be confident about what you are doing. Playing with diabetes will help you get there. It helps you learn how new activities will change your blood sugars. So even if something happens that you can't control, you at least have a good idea of what that will mean for your blood sugars.

Gone Fishing

Johnny has type 1 diabetes. He uses an insulin pump, but never paid close attention to his diabetes. The pump worked well enough to get his A1c down to 7.5%.

During an appointment, he told his doctor about an upcoming fishing trip. His doctor replied that all that extra activity would put him at risk for low blood sugars. He advised Johnny to tell his friends about his diabetes so that they could take action. Then Johnny explained that he was going alone. His doctor told him it was not safe, especially following his recent history of low blood sugars. Johnny and said he was going anyway. His wife asked if she could go along, and he said she could stay on the beach if she wanted.

The morning of his trip, Johnny walked out of the house with his insulin pump, meter, regular soda (for lows), beer, and a cell phone. When he got on the boat, he realized he forgot his meter in the car. He decided it was too late to go back now. At his fishing spot, he ate to keep his blood sugar up. The sun came out and he started sweating. Then a fish bit on the line. He stood up, excited, and his legs buckled. He fell overboard and struggled in the water, his head suddenly cloudy. He heard his wife shouting from the shore and started swimming towards her. She dove in, swimming as fast she could to meet him. Together, they struggled to the beach, drenched and exhausted.

Johnny's blood sugar was 42 mg/dL (2.3 mmol/L). Johnny wondered what would have happened if he had been truly alone.

....

Johnny only wanted to do something for himself, by himself. But diabetes comes with extra responsibilities. He had put himself in a situation where he could have become dehydrated, developed low blood sugar and not known it, and where he had no support. He was doing things he wasn't used to doing, in a place he was unfamiliar with. He had put himself and his wife in danger.

As you play with your diabetes, it is important to err on the side of safety. This is never truer than when you are doing things outside of your normal routines. When things change, your risk of unanticipated problems multiplies. When all else fails, sometimes you need to think outside the box, as Jason's story illustrates.

....

Desert High

Jason and his bride, Stella, were driving from Las Vegas to Los Angeles when they stopped in one of the small cafes that pop up on well-traveled desert highways. After lunch, Jason opened his diabetes bag and realized he had forgotten all of his medication. He groaned, turned to Stella, and said, "Oh, no. What now?"

Jason checked his blood sugars, thankful that he at least had his meter. His blood sugar was over 180 mg/dL (10 mmol/L) and he just finished eating. It would only go up from here. He racked his brain for options. There wasn't a pharmacy within 100 miles, and he wanted to get his sugars down before driving.

Jason took Stella by the arm. "Honey, would you like to take an emergency walk with me?" Jason had always relied on exercise for lowering his blood sugars and now seemed like the perfect time to get moving. Together, they spent the next hour walking around outside the café. He was tired and sweaty, but didn't feel too terribly. He stopped and checked his blood sugar. He was at 195 mg/dL (10.8 mmol/L). His blood sugar wasn't at his goal, but considering that it had barely risen in the hour after his meal, he was pretty satisfied. But he wasn't sure he was ready to drive.

Jason drank some water, took a 15-minute break, and then continued walking for another forty minutes. Now his blood sugar had dropped to 170 mg/dL (9.4 mmol/L). He felt pretty good and knew the exercise would continue to work his sugar down in the hours to follow. He was past the peak blood sugar in his meal, and it would only get better.

....

PUT LESS EFFORT INTO DIABETES

At first glance, this headline may seem like an oxymoron, but it's in sync with the idea of using natural rhythms to make diabetes more predictable. In his book *Thinking, Fast and Slow*, Daniel Kahneman writes about the two systems our brains use to process information.[30] The first works on an intuitive level. This is the part of your brain that helps you recognize a face, brush your teeth without thinking about it, or floats the feeling that you ought to avoid a dark alley. It's built on instincts and habits.

The second system is the rational one, the part of the brain you use to figure out a complex math problem, choose a car, or navigate a new city. This part of your brain can handle complex tasks, but requires far more effort to engage. You must direct your attention to use it.

These two systems work together. The intuitive mind feeds ideas and intuitions to your rational mind. The rational mind processes this information, especially new information, and decides what to do with it. If your rational system consistently comes to the same decision, it can form into a habit and take less effort in the future.

This concept has a lot of implications for people with diabetes. When you are first diagnosed and start checking your blood sugars, you may question whether the numbers on your meter are reliable enough to merit taking medication. You may question how much medication you should take. Your intuitive mind is full of fears and concerns, while your rational mind is overwhelmed by the amount of decisions to make and the limited information you have to make them. Both systems are overtaxed.

Food is especially challenging. You have a lifetime of intuitive thoughts about food. Is an apple healthy or unhealthy? What about a baked potato? Suddenly, your rational mind is in an intense and ongoing discussion with your intuitive mind. This is stressful, especially if you don't want to be thinking about these things in the first place.

Eventually, with practice, this becomes easier. The decisions that you make slowly become habits. Rather than employing your rational mind to decide if a food will impact your blood sugars, you begin to employ your intuitive mind. Eating a pickle becomes a stress-free experience. Your intuitive mind knows that it's been okay in the past and is not concerned. Your rational mind sees no reason to object. You eat and enjoy your pickle.

The challenge is when the situation changes; the intuitive mind says something is okay, and the rational mind does not object. For example, you visit the doctor and he diagnoses you with hypertension. Suddenly, you need to watch your salt intake. The pickle that was fine for the last forty years is now something you need to think about. But the intuitive mind doesn't make a fuss, and the rational mind doesn't notice (or want) to object.

There is a middle ground between letting your intuitive mind run on autopilot and justifying every decision that you make. Returning to our pickle, it might mean lowering the stakes of eating a pickle. Rather than buying whole pickles, you start buying ones that have been quartered. You know that you can snack on one of those without risk to your blood pressure.

Rely on Your Intuition

In the beginning, you constantly use your rational mind to evaluate your choices. Through practice, this process becomes more intuitive. It takes less effort.

But as you get more comfortable, thriving with diabetes requires you to employ your rational mind strategically. To minimize the impact of diabetes, you must be able to recognize bumps in the road before you hit them and quickly troubleshoot when you do. This is why we spend so much time talking about diabetes confounders in this book. That is a simple checklist of things that can cause your intuitive approach to diabetes to fail. When you have a confounder, the normal relationships between cause and effect break down, and your rational mind must decide on a different approach.

We want to help you make diabetes as easy as possible. It shouldn't be something you have to think about 24/7. We want your intuitive mind to take ownership of most of the decisions. At the same time, we have provided tools and a process for knowing when your rational mind needs to take over as well as simple ways it can figure out the solutions to the problem that you are facing.

We also want you to feel good about how you manage your diabetes. Your intuitive mind is comfortable with the approach, and your rational mind is not protesting. It is important to recognize when the intuitive and rational minds are in conflict. Identify the source of that conflict and find a way to resolve it.

When you find the right balance between intuitive and rational thinking, you are in a place of thriving. With practice, your mind has learned to intuitively navigate the routines that make up your days. You can even recognize the presence of confounders and employ your rational mind to solve them. The more you safely manage diabetes intuitively, the more your rational mind can focus on living your life the way you want.

GO FROM GOOD TO GREAT

So far in this book, we have focused on skills and strategies to get your blood sugars into your target range and keep them there. Some people want to go beyond the usual goals to achieve more normal blood sugars. There is incomplete research on the advantages of going beyond the medical targets. This is especially true because aiming for low targets can mean higher risk of low blood sugars. In this section, we will look at tools that you can use to fine-tune your management of blood sugar trends.

Look at Time in Range Instead of A1c

The phrase "time in range" means that rather than focusing on your average blood sugars or A1c, you are looking at how much of your day is spent inside your target range. This is a very new concept. Before continuous glucose meters, it was impossible to know how much time you spent in your target range.

Why look at time in range? Recent studies have shown that there are major flaws to relying on A1c as the sole measurement. The following charts, for example, show how different people can be with the same A1c result of 7%. They are each aiming for blood sugars around 80 mg/dL to 100 mg/dL (4.4 mmol/L to 5.6 mmol/L) with increases below 180 mg/dL (10 mmol/L) after meals.

John (figure 7.1) spends most of his day with blood sugars nicely in his target range and experiences mild and less frequent low blood sugars.

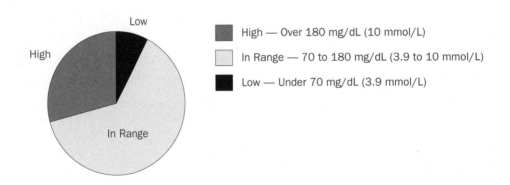

FIGURE 7.1 John has an A1c of 7% and spends much of his day in range.

Mary (figure 7.2), on the other hand, experiences frequent and severe low blood sugars followed by frequent and severe high blood sugars.

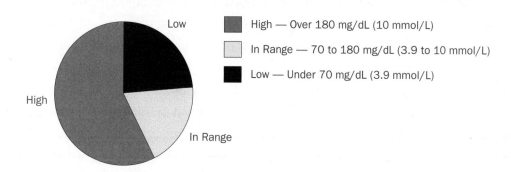

FIGURE 7.2 Mary has an A1c of 7% and spends all day on a blood sugar roller coaster.

Now, one very lucky person (figure 7.3) spends all day in their target range without any lows and any highs.

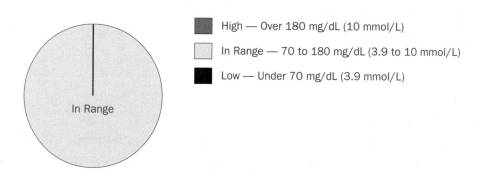

FIGURE 7.3 One lucky person has no lows or highs and still has an A1c of 7%.

John, Mary, and our hypothetical lucky person all have an A1c of 7%. Yet, their experiences are dramatically different. While John feels pretty good most of the time,

Mary is stuck on an awful roller coaster of highs and lows. How is it possible that they both have the same A1c?

Remember that the A1c is an approximate average of your blood sugars. Someone who has frequent lows and highs can achieve the same A1c as someone who has more stable blood sugars. If you are getting a lower A1c at the expense of hopping on a blood sugar roller coaster, it's not worth it. All those high blood sugars are still causing the silent changes that contribute to complications, and the A1c could be hiding it.

This is a key reason why it's important to be smart about the medical recommendations to achieve an A1c of 6.5% (the current target recommended by most). If you have other confounders that make diabetes management more challenging than usual, the only way to get there may be taking too much medication, which more often than not causes roller coaster blood sugars. The major medical organizations that suggest these targets all recognize that they must be achieved safely or they are not appropriate for you.

Because continuous glucose meters are so new, we have very little research on how "time in range" affects your risk of long-term complications, which can take many years or even decades for complications to appear. Studies suggest that reducing swings in blood sugars—even with higher average blood sugar—is better than having frequent highs followed by lows. The takeaway is to limit wild swings in blood sugars as much as possible and spend more time safely in range.

LIMIT AFTER-MEAL HIGHS

As you get closer to your target range, blood sugar increases after meals will have more and more influence on your A1c than pre-meal sugars. One study found that when you have an A1c of around 6%, over 80 percent of that number is determined by your post-meal blood sugars. However, in someone with an A1c of 9%, only 40 percent was due to post-meal numbers.[31]

Other studies have shown that your post-meal blood sugars are connected to your risk of heart problems. They are even more important than your blood sugars upon waking. For most meals, the peak blood sugar is 60 to 90 minutes after you start eating and then lowering back towards your target range over a period of two or three hours. If your doctor advises you to check one hour after a meal, he is looking at how high your sugars get. If they recommend checking three or four hours after the meal, they are looking at how effectively your treatment can bring them back to target before the next meal.

There are two basic strategies for lowering the blood sugar spike of a certain amount of carbohydrates after meals. First, you can slow down digestion of your food so your insulin, whether injected or natural, has more time to work. Second, you can make your insulin work faster.

Slow Down Your Digestion

- **Change the Content of Your Meals.** One easy option is to reduce the total number of carbohydrates. The second is to look at the type of carbohydrates you are eating. One imperfect measure of how much a food will increase your blood sugars is called the Glycemic Index (GI). The GI is basically a measure of how much a food raises your blood sugars during the first two hours after you eat, compared to other foods. It is rated on a 100-point scale, with 1 as the lowest impact and 100 as the highest (eating pure glucose). Here are some examples:

- **Low GI Foods— under 55 points:** beans (white, black, pink, kidney, lentil, soy, almond, peanut, walnut, and chickpea); small seeds (sunflower, flax, pumpkin, poppy, and sesame); most whole grains (oat, rye, and barley); most vegetables; most sweet fruits (peaches, strawberries, and mangoes); and fructose

- **Medium GI Foods—56 to 69 points:** whole wheat, pita bread, basmati rice, unpeeled boiled potato, grape juice, raisins, prunes, pumpernickel bread, cranberry juice, regular ice cream, sucrose, and bananas

- **High GI Foods—70 points and above:** white bread, most white rice, corn flakes, most breakfast cereals, potato, pretzels, parsnip, and bagels

You may have noticed that fruits are lower on the Glycemic Index. However, consider the quantities that you eat. Multiple servings of a low GI food will still spike your blood sugar. For example, 10 grams of carbohydrates from sweet fruits may raise your blood sugars more slowly than pretzels. However, because a handful of sweet fruits are denser with carbs than a handful of pretzels, you may likely see a bigger increase in blood sugars from the fruit. It is important to look at the total carbohydrates you consume and not just the GI.

- **Split the Meal.** If you eat all of your carbohydrates at once, it is more challenging for your body to process them. One option is to split your meals in half. For example, you could postpone dessert and enjoy it after your post-dinner walk. If you have a flexible work environment, you could eat part of your lunch at lunchtime and part as an early afternoon snack.

- **Increase Post-Meal Physical Activity.** When you're active, blood goes away from your stomach and to your muscles, slowing down digestion. For this to be effective, you must start moving within thirty minutes of your meal.

- **Consider Medications That Slow Digestion.** Refer back to Chapter 3 on medications and look at DPP-4s and GLP-1s in particular.

Speed Up Your Insulin

- **Increase Post-Meal Activity.** Exercise not only increases blood flow to your muscles, but it also helps them absorb insulin better. For many hours after you are active, your body will use insulin more efficiently. In one study, just 30 minutes of very slow walking reduced the average spike by 30 mg/dL (1.7 mmol/L). The post-meal blood sugar peaks were 45% higher when participants did not walk.[31]

- **Choose the Right Mealtime Insulin.** If you are using regular insulin (Humulin R or Novolin R) at meal times, talk to your doctor about switching to analog insulin (Humalog, Novolog, or Apidra). Regular insulins have a peak at two to three hours and last for four to six hours. The newer analog insulins have a much faster peak of around one hour and last three to four hours. This makes it easier to match them to mealtime increases.

- **Take Insulin 15 to 30 Minutes Before the Meal.** Rapid-acting insulin is only rapid compared to the older injected insulin. Even rapid insulin takes 15 minutes to start working. One study concluded that taking rapid-acting insulin twenty minutes prior to a meal resulted in significantly better blood sugars than when it was taken at the start of the meal or twenty minutes into it.[18, 19]

- **Be Careful When Taking Insulin Before a Meal.** When injecting insulin before a meal, it's extremely important to watch out for low blood sugars (see The Pizza Challenge on page 119). This can be an especially big problem if you can't control when your food will be served. You don't want to inject insulin and then get stuck waiting on a slow restaurant kitchen.

TAKE CARE WITH NPH INSULIN

NPH insulin is often prescribed because it's less expensive than other insulin. However, it starts working more slowly than regular or analog insulins and is not very effective at covering higher blood sugars from meals. Because NPH works over a much longer period than these insulins, it tends to work inconsistently from one injection to another. When mixed with another rapid-acting insulin, you'll find it becomes even harder to manage the peaks. If your physician recommends NPH insulin or an insulin mixture containing NPH insulin, make sure you get specific instructions of how he or she wants you to use it in relation to your daily meals and activity.

EMBRACE EXERCISE

The usual warnings about strenuous exercise apply even more to people with diabetes. First, it's important to consult a doctor when starting a new exercise program to ensure that there are no underlying physical problems that could hurt you. As we discussed before, if you find that mild exercise is increasing your blood sugars, talk to your doctor about it and consider requesting a heart stress test.

If you haven't exercised in recent memory, be careful to start slowly. You are at a heightened risk for injury when getting started. It can take several months or more for the body to adapt to increased physical activity. If you have an ambitious goal like running a marathon, those adaptations can take a year or more to do safely.

Changing your body's ability to lose weight will take about a few weeks to start. The weight that you lose in the first few weeks has to do with water loss. When you hit a wall and seem to stop losing weight, this is when your body starts making the changes it needs to start losing the extra fat.

Remember, to lose weight, your need for insulin has to decrease. So long as you have excess insulin in your body, it is physiologically impossible for your cells to release fat. (Excess insulin can enhance both muscle growth and fat storage. If you are consuming more calories than you need and your muscles aren't growing, then your fat cells are.)

As you get in better shape, your body can use more sugar as fuel without requiring insulin. As we mentioned earlier, our muscle cells have two different pathways for accessing sugar. One requires insulin and the other does not. As you continue to exercise, the number of pathways not requiring insulin expands.

Exercise, especially prolonged exercise, can continue to lower blood sugars for more than 24 hours. This is a good thing, but you need to pay attention to avoid low blood sugar if you take either insulin or sulfonylureas. These medicines cause your body to put insulin into your body without regard for your blood sugar levels.

If you take insulin, don't take injections into your limbs while exercising. Your body will use insulin much faster than if it's injected into your abdomen.

Now, start playing!

PART 3

THRIVE
FOR LIFE

"Between stimulus and response there is a space. In that space is our power to choose our response. In our response lies our growth and our freedom."

—Viktor Frankl

Chapter 8

Lead Your Health Care Team

The ability to live with diabetes has improved dramatically over the last 125 years. An 1884 medical text paints a grim picture of living with diabetes before insulin:

> *As the disease advances he becomes listless and debilitated, and there is decrease or abolition of sexual desire; in women the menses are often suppressed. The tongue is red or coated, and nearly always thicker than normal; the gums are pale, retracted, and bleed easily, and the teeth become carious. There are nausea and vomiting … with constipation and most patients complain of a constant sinking feeling in the [stomach].*
>
> *It gets worse. High blood sugars increasingly defeated the body, leading to a slow but inevitable death.*

After the discovery of insulin in 1921, patients and doctors overcame the worst of these symptoms. Dr. Elliott Joslin, considered the first great diabetes doctor in the United States, writes in the 1937 edition of *Diabetic Manual* that "Insulin rescued the diabetic and set him on his feet."[32]

With insulin, short-term complications, while extremely difficult, are less devastating: "thirst, hunger, and the passage of increased quantities of urine with loss of weight and strength. Itching of the skin, particularly about the genitals, is common."[33]

Soon, Dr. Joslin is full of hope—under one condition. "It is perfectly true that diabetes is a chronic disease, but unlike rheumatism and cancer, it is painless; unlike tuberculosis, it is clean and not contagious, and in contrast to many diseases of the skin, it is not unsightly. Moreover, it is susceptible to treatment, and the downward course of a patient can be promptly checked. Treatment, however, rests in the hands of the patient."[32]

In the 1970s, with the ability to check blood sugars at home, the possibility of people with diabetes caring for themselves improved dramatically. Suddenly, it wasn't a matter of getting a prescription for a fixed diet and guessing the right amount of medication. It was now possible for someone to peek inside their blood and start influencing their actual blood sugars. The last twenty years has brought a dramatic increase in life expectancy for those living with diabetes.

SELF CARE VS. YOUR DOCTORS' GOALS

Working effectively with your health care team can present real challenges. Do you have trouble remembering all of the instructions when you get home? Do you question whether your doctor really knows best? Are you concerned about the safety of your medication or so frustrated by its side effects that you want to skip it altogether? Are you being asked to make changes that, deep down, you know you won't really make? Do you know the best times to check your blood sugars and what to do with the information? Are you comfortable working with numbers?

LIMIT THE LOWS FOR LIVELY DAYS!

High blood sugars are a major focus in managing diabetes. Yet, one of the biggest dangers is low blood sugars, especially when unrecognized. Read more in Chapter 5: Step 2: Limit the Lows (page 83).

The advice you need is often too complex to convey in a few short visits per year. Diabetes is not simple and too many things change from day to day and from hour to hour to fix it all with a single medication, a change in a particular meal, or a little bit more exercise. You may leave your doctor and be unsure about what to do next. You may have questions that you don't know how to ask or feel uncomfortable asking. In such short visits, far too much goes unaddressed.

A PERSONAL CHECKLIST

Did you ever think diabetes was "child's play"? Meet Kathy Sue.

Kathy Sue was diagnosed with type 1 diabetes when she was five years old. A strong-willed little girl, she decided that diabetes was not going to run her life. As a child, she played with her diabetes, seeing how everything from ice cream to jumping changed her blood sugars.

She never told her mother or her father. Kathy Sue was also careful not to tell her doctor because she figured Dr. Ann would shout at her if she did. Kathy Sue thought adults took diabetes way too seriously.

The good thing was that she discovered a lot when she played with her diabetes. For instance, food was not the only thing that caused her sugar levels to change. Many years later, the grown up Kathy Sue shared her list of *Eight Things That Predict My Sugars* with her family doctor:

- Not getting enough sleep
- Stress from the kids
- Pain (like when I broke my ankle last winter)
- Just sitting around and snacking on stuff
- A fever
- Chopping wood, especially in the late afternoon
- Cleaning the house
- Breastfeeding the twins (I love them, but I'm glad I don't have to do that again!)

Kathy Sue's doctor smiled and went on with the appointment. He said it was interesting but there were other things he needed to address. She was furious. She demanded that their family switch doctors.

"Why did he do that?" she asked, practically screaming at her husband, Doug. "Dr. Ned should know better!"

"Maybe Dr. Ned has his other things on his mind."

Doug was right.

Your Doctor's Checklist

When a doctor sees a patient with diabetes, he has some things on his mind that he has to address. It's an important list, although a number of things important to Kathy Sue and you are not on it. Your doctor's checklist may look something like this:

- How regularly do you take your medication? When?
- What is your Hemoglobin A1c?
- Did you get an eye exam during the past year?
- Is kidney function normal and stable? Is there protein in your urine?
- Are your blood pressure, heart rate, and heart rhythm normal?
- Are your lipid levels satisfactory?
- Did your weight change since your last visit?
- When did you have your feet checked last?

- Do you have any numbness, tingling, or pain in your hands or feet?
- Are you following an appropriate diet?
- Are you meeting the guidelines for physical exercise?
- Do you smoke cigarettes?

Your doctor is expected to create a medical history that covers all aspects of your health, including any hospital stays, emergency room visits, or surgeries, as well as any changes in health status or medication. Medicines should be reviewed one by one. Your doctor should look at the labels on the bottles, review how each medication is taken, and even what pharmacy you use.

This may sound like an overemphasis on reviewing medication, but it's necessary. When doctors ask patients about their medications two or three times in a visit, they often get different answers about how the medications are taken. This is especially common in older patients. Taking incorrect doses of medication can have dangerous consequences.

All the items on the doctor's checklist are important. In fact, this checklist is primarily what your doctor is paid to do. In the United States, each year the National Committee for Quality Assurance (NCQA) looks at conditions like diabetes and what is required to deliver high-quality care. It publishes guidelines called Health Effectiveness Data and Information Sets (HEDIS). Insurance companies and government agencies use these guidelines to determine what they will pay for. Other countries have similar processes. If what your doctor does during your visit isn't on the guidelines, the practice might not get paid. The HEDIS guideline for adult diabetes tells your doctor to evaluate the following:

- Hemoglobin A1c
- LDL cholesterol levels
- Retinal eye examination
- Tests for kidney changes and early signs of abnormal kidney function
- Abnormal blood pressure

Let's quickly review each of these measures.

Hemoglobin A1c

Often shortened to HbA1c or just A1c, this measures glucose binding to red blood cell hemoglobin. Because red blood cells live for three to four months, the A1c gives us an estimate of average blood sugars during the three previous months. Target levels of hemoglobin A1c are usually 6.5%. Higher levels are associated with increased incidence of heart attacks and strokes.[9] Maintaining target A1cs can delay complications and extend life.[10]

LDL Cholesterol

This is the "bad" cholesterol that, when elevated, is associated with heart attacks and cardiac death. The risk of heart disease is three times higher in people with diabetes. If the person with diabetes smokes, the risk of heart disease is a startling 11 times higher. Efforts to reduce LDL cholesterol have contributed to a decrease in deaths from heart disease and stroke in people with diabetes.[34]

Retinal Eye Exams

Examinations by an eye doctor (ophthalmologist or optometrist) may reveal early blood vessel changes in the eyes. Blindness can be caused when new blood vessels form in the eyes, resulting in bleeding, swelling, or scarring. This blindness is preventable for most people with early detection and treatment of diabetic eye changes.[35]

Kidney Health

Blood and urine testing can detect kidney disease in people with diabetes. Early treatment can prevent or delay kidney failure and the need for hemodialysis or kidney transplants.[36]

Blood Pressure

Keeping your blood pressure in a recommended range of 140/90 or less is vital to preventing strokes, heart attacks, and kidney failure in people with diabetes. When you have hypertension for months or years, blood vessel changes are often not reversible and can lead to disability and death.[9]

Going Forward

All of these measurements are signs that the doctor has been thorough in his evaluation. They also serve as useful ways to measure your progress. When these numbers improve, a wealth of research shows your long-term health improves, too.

Like Kathy Sue's husband suggested, Dr. Ned has very good reasons for his checklist. However, you have very good reasons for your checklist, too. The rest of this book will show you how to satisfy the needs on your checklist. You will need to be assertive to ensure that all of your needs are addressed, not just the ones on your doctor's list.

YOUR HEALTH CARE TEAM

It is a challenge to figure out how to get all the tools of diabetes management to work together. This requires a lot of technical expertise that can only be provided by trained health care providers. Yet, far too many people feel that their doctor does not listen to or understand them.

In thousands of conversations with people living with diabetes, we have heard this frustration bubble to the surface. To be fair, the people who are focused on reforming our health care system know this and have been struggling to find a way to improve the doctor-patient relationship.

Get Your Doc's Attention with "Teach Back"

There is a strategy you can use to gain a voice in the doctor's office. This has been proven effective and is being widely taught to doctors as a tool for improving health outcomes. It's called teach back.[37] The idea is simple: you explain back to the doctor what he has suggested that you do. This ensures you understand what was said, are in agreement, and are able to do it. Here are some ways to start the conversation with your doctor.

- "We covered a lot today. Let me see if I can summarize what I need to do."
- "You have prescribed metformin. Let me make sure I understand why and when I'm taking it."
- "So if I understand this correctly, when I get home, I'm going to…"

The simple act of repeating back your understanding of the conversation ensures that you and your doctor are on the same page. If there is something you know you are not going to do, this also gives you a place to share that. "Doctor, as I understand you, I am to take a shot before my meals. But I am not comfortable taking insulin at work and see that being a problem."

If you are going to lead your health care team, you must speak up. It starts here. Your health care team is there to serve your needs. If you leave with an unsustainable plan or one you don't really understand, the only person who loses is you.

Doctors

The doctor has two roles in helping you manage your diabetes. The first role is to diagnose and treat medical problems. These can be immediate, such as a high blood sugar, or long-term, like preventing complications. The doctor works in the examination room or the hospital to treat illness by taking a history, doing a physical exam, checking your medications and adjusting them, and monitoring for diabetes complications.

Your doctor's second role is to orchestrate the other members of your medical support team around your care. You should be able to call on your doctor and this team to connect you with the medical resources that you need to be healthy.

In busy and complex health care systems, your doctor in the examining room or in the hospital may not be the same doctor who answers when you call with an urgent problem three weeks later. The responsibility of orchestrating your medical care then ends up on your shoulders, not on the doctor who you saw previously.

It is important to have a discussion with your doctor about the team before you walk out of the examination room. Who should you call with problems? Who else might be involved in your care? The information could prevent a trip to an emergency room.

Nurses, Nurse Practitioners, and Physician's Assistants

Every health care environment includes people who help support the patient and facilitate communication with the doctor as needed. This group can include physician's assistants, nurses, and nurse practitioners who have more specialized training. Doctors, especially diabetes doctors, are often pulled in many different directions. Their support staff can make sure they are pulled in yours. Traditionally, only a doctor can write a prescription, although increasing numbers of nurse practitioners and physician's assistants can, too. Regardless, anyone in your doctor's office can facilitate updating your prescriptions. These supporters can also show you how to use your meter, give you more information about the tools you are using, and give you an opportunity to talk about issues you haven't had a chance to bring up with your doctor.

Dietitian

An accurate understanding of how food impacts diabetes is essential. At the same time, making food choices that are consistent with your tastes and lifestyle is critical if you want to sustain your success over the long term. A dietitian can help you with both of these things. A dietitian can teach you how to count the carbohydrates and maintain your nutrition. A dietitian can also be very helpful in adjusting your diet for weight loss, if that is one of your goals.

This is an especially important area for you to take charge. Bring a diary of your food and what you eat. If your dietitian makes recommendations, make sure they are consistent with the types of foods that you and your family like to eat. If you're not getting joy from your diet, you will not stick with it. If your dietitian is not familiar with your food culture, you may want to look for one who understands you better, or is willing to learn.

Certified Diabetes Educators (CDE)

Your health plan likely gives you access to a health care professional called a Certified Diabetes Educator (CDE) who has spent years training and working in the field of diabetes. You can work with a CDE to get your questions answered during extended, uninterrupted periods of time. For example, how do you keep a food diary? How do you count carbohydrates? How do you operate your meter? This is your chance to get an excellent understanding of the fundamental topics of diabetes. CDEs have a wealth of experience and insight to share about how to put this information into action in your own life.

Health Care Workers

Health care workers are newer to the health care system. As it has grown in size and complexity, the need for advocates that can help patients navigate effectively has grown too. If you are in a large practice or hospital system, you may find that there is a health care worker available on site. More typically, you can find them among community or religious organizations.

A health care worker can be especially helpful in overcoming obstacles like language, culture, and familiarity with payment systems. If you need extra help navigating the health care system, ask someone at your doctor's office or hospital if they can recommend a health care worker to assist you.

Family, Friends, and Peers

The people around you have an enormous impact on your ability to manage diabetes. This influence may range from the food that your loved ones cook to whether or not your friends drag you out to a new restaurant or a hike in the woods.

As you build your health care team, think carefully about the role of the people that are currently around you, whether family, friends or co-workers, as well as those that you would like to have support from. For example, there are many great online resources where you can meet other people dealing with the same issues as you. There may also be more structured local support groups.

Your peers with diabetes can be especially effective at helping you solve problems, acquire and understand useful information, and provide ongoing emotional support.

Chapter 9

Change Your Habits

Habits are things that you do automatically without thinking. Sometimes, you are consciously aware of your habits. Other times, you are guided by the invisible hands of instinct or social pressures.

The strength of habits is that they don't require much effort and are easy to do. The downside is that changing automatic behaviors can be difficult, though it becomes easier when you understand how habits change. The really good news is that if you adopt new, more productive habits, they will soon be as effortless as the less-than-useful ones they are replacing. So how do habits work? And how do you decide which ones are worth changing?

The last two decades has seen a wealth of research on how we form habits and can change them. In *The Power of Habit: Why We Do What We Do in Life and Business*, author Charles Duhigg outlines the relatively simple process:[38] You encounter a cue that triggers you to perform a routine, and you get a reward. This reward can be small. When you brush your teeth, it can be the feeling of cleanliness and lessening your fear of cavities. It is not necessarily healthy. With a cigarette, the reward can be satisfying your body's craving for nicotine. For a gambler, it's the flood of endorphins that come with a periodic win.

In this chapter, we will look at some of the ways that you can change your habits. But first, let's take a look at the most obvious—yet unreliable—way to change your behavior: practicing self-control.

WHY YOU CAN'T RELY ON SELF-CONTROL

In 1996, a team of researchers led by Roy Baumeister was on the cusp of uncovering a surprising fact about limits of self-control.[39] The experiment began by putting participants in a room in which the air smelled of freshly baked cookies. Some of the participants were invited to enjoy a few chocolate chip cookies. The others were required to eat the antithesis of a chocolate chip cookie: a bunch of radishes. To make things worse, researchers asked the participants to skip the prior meal to ensure they arrived hungry. The radish group looked unhappy. Some gazed "longingly" at the chocolate chip cookies. Others picked them up and sniffed them deeply before setting them down.

The really interesting part of the study came next. Each participant was given an impossible puzzle to solve and instructed to solve it. Which group of people tried harder to solve the puzzle? Hint: it was not the radish eaters! They were spent.

Self-control is like a muscle. The more you exercise it without rest, the more it loses strength, until it finally fails. If you spend an hour focusing on one task, then when you move to the next, you are at a disadvantage unless you rest in between the two tasks. Eventually you seem to run out of gas.

This study and others transformed how we look at self-control. If your environment is stacked against you, you will use up your strong drive for self-control, and despite good intentions, your efforts may fail. This can lead to undesirable food choices like late-night binge eating or skipping your exercise plans.

Meanwhile, thinking positive thoughts about ourselves can dramatically increase our self-control. If you believe you have more self-control, then you actually have more self-control.[40] There are many examples of people making dramatic and long-lasting life changes. These feats of self-control are real and inspiring.

There are two key lessons here. First, it's important to give yourself breaks from practicing self-control. If you keep your self-control muscle engaged all of the time, eventually it will give out and lead you to decisions you will later regret.

Second, change your environment to reduce your need for self-control. Schedule time to do effortless activities, whether a coffee break, chatting with a friend, playing the piano, or reading a magazine, and be sure to avoid starving yourself during the day. The radish experiment would have been very different if there were no freshly baked cookies, and the participants had come in after a good lunch.

CHANGE YOUR ENVIRONMENT

All of your habits are triggered by some stimulus in your environment. In the chocolate chip cookie experiment, it was the smell and sight of the cookies that triggered the participants' desire to eat them. If there had been no cookies, most of the participants would have cheerfully attempted to solve the puzzles without much thought about food.

Your day is full of such triggers. When you wake up in the morning and enter the bathroom, what do you do first? Do you brush your teeth? Turn on the shower? We spend about 40 percent of our days acting out of habit, each one triggered by cues in our environment.

Triggers can have a powerful effect on your mood. After all, chocolate chip cookies don't just put a sweet taste in your mind; they may bring back the childhood image of Grandma's freshly baked and gooey chocolate cookies in your mind. Radishes just can't compete.

So how can you use this knowledge of triggers to change your habits? If you eat snacks often, you could put out a plate of healthier options in the place where you had a plate of cookies.

Take Rita. She was committed to eating healthier lunches at work, but was often in a rush and ended up snacking from the vending machine or going out to grab lunch with friends. Finally, she figured out a strategy to change her habits.

....

Note to Self!

My workweek is extremely busy. Between my husband, children, and work, I don't have a lot of time to prepare healthy lunches. I don't have enough energy at night or time in the mornings.

I do have some time on Sundays.

I decided that I was going to cook a healthy meal with lots of leftovers every Sunday night. Then I would bring those leftovers the first few days of the week. As a reward to myself, I went out and got a new set of storage containers and threw out all of the mismatched ones we had. The new ones were microwave safe and had multiple compartments. When I filled them up with my first big batch of leftovers, I put a little sticky note on each one, "Mom's Lunch Monday" and "Mom's Lunch Tuesday", and placed them in the fridge.

The very first Monday, I forgot my lunch. My daughter woke up late, and I rushed out the door without thinking about lunch. When I got home that night, I put a sticky note on the garage door that said, "Remember Your Lunch!" For good measure, I put a second one on my car window. I was not going to forget again.

....

David shared the story of how he adjusted triggers in his environment to start exercising.

....

Suited Up

I wanted to start running, but it wasn't going very well. Looking over my schedule, I quickly realized that I only had time to run in the morning. But I'm not much of a morning person, and it wasn't working. I would constantly hit the snooze button until it was too late. I started getting frustrated with myself. A friend suggested that I make it as easy as possible to run in the morning. She told me to put my running shoes next to the bed with the socks out. She suggested that I sleep in my running shorts. It seemed like a silly little thing, but I decided to give it a try.

The next morning, the alarm went off and I forced myself to sit up. I could see my socks right in front of me. I put them on, laced up my shoes, and practically slept-walked down the stairs and out the door. Before I knew it, I had run fifteen minutes.

Over the next few months, I used this trick to great effect. Soon, whenever I woke up with my running shorts on, it would trigger me to sit up and start the process. Eventually, it barely took any effort at all to get running.

Going to sleep at a reasonable time the night before was my next challenge. That one was quite a lot harder to tackle.

....

MAKE AND EAT HEALTHY FOOD

You can also change your environment at home to make healthy food easy to eat and less healthy foods harder to eat. This means stocking your refrigerator, freezer, and pantry with healthy food options. Make these foods the easiest ones to reach. You may want to keep a bowl of nuts out on the counter, while burying cookies in the back corner of a drawer. Whatever you do, don't put the cookies on display in the middle of the counter where you will be forced to covet it as you walk by like a participant in the radish experiment.

Think about it: it only takes thirty minutes of self-control to buy healthy food at the grocery store. It takes a week of self-control not to eat something unhealthy once it is in your house.

Dining Tips for Weight Loss

If you want to lose weight, it is a good idea to change the size of the dinner plate you use. When you have a bigger plate, you tend to eat more food. In one study, people at a Super Bowl party ate 56 percent more calories when they used a larger bowl.[41] Switching from a 12 inch (30 cm) dinner plate to a 10 inch (25.4 cm) plate can have a surprising impact on how much food you eat.

You can use similar strategies when you go out to eat. First, you can decide what to order in advance. Review the menu online to choose a meal when you don't have the sights and smells of other things around to tempt you. Then, at the restaurant, be the one to order first. One study showed that your food choices are influenced by what others order before you. If you decide in advance and order first, it takes far less self-control than if you were influenced by choices made by other people at your table.

When the food arrives, ask for a take-home container and leave a reasonable portion on your plate. Over the last decades, portion sizes have soared far beyond what any normal person needs. Once you start eating, it can be very hard to stop—especially for those of us who were raised to clean our plates.

Many diabetes challenges revolve around the amounts and types of foods you eat. So it's especially important to make sure that you don't feel deprived by your food choices, especially if you find yourself binging later on unhealthy foods. It is much better to have little treats throughout the day than a major binge right before bed.

The First Time Is Usually the Hardest

Let's say you want to start cooking more meals with sautéed vegetables like spinach. If you are not very familiar with cooking spinach, you will have a lot of questions to answer:

- How do you know if the spinach you are buying is any good?
- How much should you purchase? How much does it shrink when cooking?
- What's the best way to cook it?
- How do you know when it's done cooking and ready to eat?
- Will you like the way it comes out?

Each of these unknowns is a roadblock preventing you from cooking spinach. When faced with all of these questions, isn't it easier to fall back on something you already know how to make?

The first time you choose to do a new behavior, it may be challenging. But each time you repeat it, it becomes easier. You confidently pick up a bag of spinach because you know exactly how to prepare it. You no longer need to get out a cookbook and can chat with your family while it's simmering on the stove.

Make the First Time Easy

In his Behavior Model, Stanford Professor B.J. Fogg emphasizes the importance of making a behavior easy to do.[43] If something is hard to do, it takes a lot more motivation to do it. So how can you apply this to your life? It is useful to think about simplifying any habit that you want to adopt. What is preventing you from succeeding?

Say you want to walk more in the winter. Do you have a place to go, like a gym or a nearby mall? Do you have walking shoes? Do you have warm and comfortable clothes to wear in cold weather? Do you have a friend to join you and make it more enjoyable? The first time you go for your soon-to-be-daily winter walk, it may take some planning. You may need to go to the store and get some clothing. You may need to reward yourself with some hot cocoa. But each time you do it, it becomes more familiar.

When you get started with something, it's often helpful not to think about it as a life change. Instead, think about walking five minutes every day for a week or cooking the same, simple vegetable dish every Monday night. Make sure you repeat your new habit enough for it to become something that's easy to do. Don't start with a complex new dish or lifestyle program, but instead add one simple meal to your repertoire. Instead of training for a marathon, start by walking five minutes each day. Once you have a steady habit, it's much easier to do more of it. Getting started is the hardest part—so make it as easy as possible.

Leverage Your Social Nature

Asked the most important thing you can do for your health, Dr. Roizen answered, "Get a buddy!" As Chief Wellness Officer at the Cleveland Clinic, he is deeply engaged with patient health. In the last decades, study after study has shown how behaviors are contagious. If a friend gains weight, it increases your chance of gaining weight. If a friend starts smoking, it increases your chance of smoking. On the flip side, if your friend starts exercising, you are more likely to exercise. If your friend loses weight, you are more likely to lose weight, too.

David credits a running buddy with his success in keeping moving.

Buddy Power

When Carrie suggested we run a 10K, I thought she was crazy. My longest run had been twenty minutes. By my math, a 6-mile run would take at least an hour. I really wanted to be someone who had run a 10K, so I said yes, even though I didn't really think I could do it.

We decided to run three days every week. In the beginning, I was tempted to cancel a number of times. But I knew that Carrie was excited to run, and I didn't want to disappoint her.

I came to enjoy those runs. It was a good chance to vent about the day. It was also nice to spend some time with Carrie, whom I hadn't seen very frequently in recent years. And there were dozens of times when she helped me push through the end of those runs. Had I been alone, I know I would have stopped running, even if I'd been able to get started.

In hindsight, Carrie's biggest contribution was her suggestion to get dressed for running and out on the trail. I always thought running was hard. But it turns out the hardest thing is getting out the door. Once you start moving, it's actually surprisingly easy—after the first twenty minutes—to keep going.

In Chapter 12, we'll look at how to build a support network. Remember the influence that those around you have on your behavior. Changing your social environment can be far more effective than trying to will yourself into adopting new behaviors.

Chapter 10

Manage Your Emotions

Diabetes can spark a wide range of emotions. There's the smile that comes with seeing a perfect number on the meter. There's the satisfaction of stepping on a scale and seeing a result you've worked so hard to achieve. On the other hand, there's the anger at a high blood sugar disrupting an evening. There's exhaustion that comes with years or decades of managing blood sugars.

One of the keys to *Thriving with Diabetes* is gaining the ability to work through negative emotions and cultivate positive ones. Even if you have good processes for managing the ups and downs of blood sugars, you will still experience the ups and downs of emotions around your diabetes. Managing these is no less important. In fact, it's quite the contrary. Letting negative emotions fester can have a negative impact on your diabetes, while resolving them can make blood sugar control easier.[48]

DEALING WITH UNCERTAINTY

One of the great challenges of managing diabetes is all the uncertainty. Diabetes is biologically complex. The truth is that we don't always know why blood sugars are what they are. We can't always figure out why they changed. There is a reason buried somewhere inside of our bodies, but we never truly know what it is. This uncertainty can be incredibly frustrating, but you can succeed in spite of it.[47] You don't need to know everything to be successful. You just need to know enough to be effective. You don't need to do everything perfectly. You just need to do it well enough.

Sometimes, you do everything the same, but get different results. Your blood sugars are unexpectedly high. You may wonder what caused it.

- Did you say something embarrassing, which caused a spike in adrenaline?
- Are you coming down with a cold?
- Did you eat more carbohydrates than you thought?
- Is it a combination of these things?

The exact cause doesn't matter because it is in the past. So you treat the high blood sugar and go on with your life. You pay a little more attention in the hours to follow.

- Is it possible you have a bad vial of insulin?
- Did you bang your toe on a chair last night?
- Are you dealing with a confounder?

In the hours or days to come, you pay a little more attention. But that's about it. Your life goes on. Moving forward in the face of uncertainty is one characteristic that separates those who find diabetes debilitating from those who are able to thrive.

STAY OUT OF THE RUTS

Sometimes, we get stuck in mental ruts. This can happen early on when you don't have enough knowledge to understand what's really happening. For example, some people get single-mindedly focused on food and don't think about the impact of exercise, stress, and confounders. This can also happen in more experienced people, who get in the habit of reacting in a certain way without thinking through alternative explanations for what might be happening. It can also happen when you're tired and stop looking for an explanation altogether.

Look Within

When should you dig a little deeper? When not doing so could put you in an unsafe or unhappy situation. For example, if you are getting lots of unexpected high blood sugars and ignore them, you may not notice your vial of insulin has gone bad. If you're going out for a celebratory dinner with pasta and birthday cake, a bad vial of insulin can quickly ruin your evening.

This is even truer if taking too much insulin or unpredictable physical activity may be causing severe and unexpected lows, especially if you'll be driving. When in doubt, get assistance from your doctor or nurse. The uncertainty of diabetes can be particularly daunting.

In the earliest years of working on this program, we became aware that people with diabetes have much of the information that they need to figure out what is happening with their blood sugars. The problem is there is so much information, and they don't know how to use it productively.

By reframing your thoughts to focus on those things that matter most, you can escape some of the uncertainty that surrounds blood sugar management. It becomes even easier if you can take little steps to work on a particular problem and temporarily tolerate a little more uncertainty in another area.

REFRAME YOUR THOUGHTS

Beyond uncertainty, there is a whirlwind of emotions that we all experience: sadness and happiness, anger and calmness, frustration and confusion. How can you go about taking charge of these feelings?

At the heart of modern psychology is Cognitive Behavioral Therapy (CBT). The concept is that your feelings are a result of your thought patterns, so by changing the way you think, you can change the way you feel. In this style of therapy, you work with a therapist to identify the triggers for negative thoughts and reframe them in a more positive way.

For example, it's very easy to get in the habit of self-defeating internal mono-logues. One person sees a high blood sugar on their birthday and thinks, "I am a failure! Why can't I ever get this right?" A different person in the same situation might think, "Today's my birthday. Diabetes and cake don't mix very well. But that's okay. Tomorrow is a fresh day. Now, let's get back to this party."

You can imagine the different emotions that accompany each internal dialogue.

In her excellent book *Diabetes and Wellbeing: Managing the Psychological and Emotional Challenges of Diabetes Type 1 and 2*, Dr. Jen Nash outlines a five-step CBT process for changing your thoughts.[44]

This is a strategy you can use when you find yourself stuck in emotional ruts. Something happens to trigger a cascade of internal dialogue and feelings that you want to escape. Often, you get deep into it before you even realize that it's happening. But when you notice it happening, you have an opportunity to stop and ask yourself the following:

- **Step 1:** What is the situation or event? Begin by identifying what is trigger-ing your negative thoughts. Are you reacting to a specific high blood sugar measurement? Taking an insulin injection? Thinking about how your partner is treating you? In order to change your thoughts, you must first understand when and why you are having them.

- **Step 2:** What do you tell yourself? Verbalize the thought pattern that goes through your mind. Are you telling yourself that you're a failure? Thinking that this will go on forever? Wondering why you have to deal with this and others don't?

- **Step 3:** What is happening in your body? Notice what happens to your body when you are having these thought processes. Are you feeling sad, helpless, or angry? What about physically? Are you tired? Thirsty? You can also look at your behaviors. Do your thoughts trigger you to yell at a partner? Seek out food? Lie in the dark?

- **Step 4:** Examine your thoughts: ask yourself some helpful questions. This is the key step. It's time to interrogate your thoughts. Are your thoughts true? Are they helping or hurting you? Are you thinking in "all or nothing" terms? For example, "I am a failure" or "I'll never get this right" or "I'll be unhappy forever."

- **Step 5:** Develop an alternative, balanced thought. In this last step, you focus on changing your internal conversation. Are you really a failure or are you trying your best and going through a difficult period? This is when you give yourself a reality check: "My blood sugar is high, but it's not my fault. Diabetes is hard, especially with my busy travel schedule. I am doing the best that I can right now."

Let's take a look at an example. Binging on food can have a number of different causes. Sometimes, you are hungry because you aren't eating enough during the day. Other times, it's due to boredom. In her book, Dr. Nash shares the example of Janya, who is driven to eat by her overwhelming emotions.

Once Janya identified that she was triggered by her emotional state, she looked inward to understand thoughts, feelings, and behaviors. Her mind was full of thoughts like "life is too hard," "I can't manage this," and "to hell with this diet. I deserve a treat." She recognized that these thoughts were accompanied by a fast heartbeat and negative emotions like anger and hopelessness and was reaching out for food to cope.

Now, the critical step was to challenge her thoughts. Are they really true? What would a friend say if she were advising her? Janya recognized that her life is indeed hard. On the other hand, eating all that food at night was making it harder, not easier. Though she didn't feel like she could manage all of this, she was thrilled to be a mom and generally content with her job. And, once she started reflecting, she really did feel like she deserved a treat. So she looked for a way to treat herself that wouldn't make her feel guilty, like a long bubble bath and a movie.

Your thoughts won't transform themselves overnight. Simply recognizing your thoughts as they happen is a major step in the right direction. You may frequently fall back into your undesired habits, and this is okay. Don't beat yourself up. Cultivate self-awareness and move forward slowly. Thoughts can be stubborn things.

OVERCOME GUILT AND SHAME

A couple of common emotions, especially with type 2 diabetes, are guilt and shame. Guilt is an emotion that may arise when you feel like you have caused harm. Shame is when you feel the judgment of others for something that you have done wrong. They often go hand in hand. People sometimes feel like their diabetes is their own doing.

The challenge with guilt and shame is that there is often some truth beneath the surface. If your food and exercise habits contributed to weight gain and your diabetes diagnosis, then you may feel some responsibility. But if you step back, you will see that diabetes is more complex than that.

Many things contribute to a type 2 diabetes diagnosis. In spite of its association with weight, type 2 diabetes is a strongly genetic condition.[45] The fact is that most people who are obese will never develop diabetes. Yet, there are millions who have a healthy weight or are underweight and develop type 2 diabetes.

Then there are all the factors out of your control. Did you grow up in a house that encouraged unhealthy eating habits? Do you work a stressful and sedentary job that leaves you little time for physical activity? Do you live in an area without easy access to affordable and healthy food? Do you suffer from an injury that makes physical activity difficult? If you are experiencing guilt or shame over your diagnosis, it's important to recognize the factors over which you had control and those you did not.

In the case of a diabetes diagnosis, guilt can come not just from feeling like you let yourself down, but also that you are having a negative impact on your loved ones. Perhaps you can be one of the many who use diabetes as a tool for transforming their own lives in positive ways.

Forgiving yourself is an ongoing process. You can't change the past, but when you have taken appropriate responsibility and done what you can to make amends, accept yourself as you are.

ADOPT A FLOURISHING MINDSET

There is one especially powerful way to reframe the way you look at yourself and your diabetes. Riva Greenberg, an author and health coach who lives with type 1 diabetes, has developed an approach called "flourishing."

"In chronic illness we talk about 'coping,'" says Greenberg. "Yet coping depicts struggle, not doing well. Coping, as a strategy for living with diabetes, focuses on what's not working and then tries to fix those things. Conversely, a flourishing approach shifts your attention to what is already working and highlights your strengths. In addition, your focus is on what you want, a healthy, happy life, not on what you don't want, complications. You move from seeing perceived loss to what might be gained. You don't beat yourself up for mistakes, but appreciate your efforts."

This is the emotional health equivalent of Use Your Best to Fix the Rest! Accept your successes and work on expanding them. Greenberg explains:

> *In essence, you are writing a new narrative for yourself—life anew with diabetes, living and managing it well. Living from a flourishing mindset fosters strength, capability, hope, and possibilities. From this place you*

very naturally manage diabetes better. I am also helping health-professionals work from this approach.

I recognized flourishing ten years ago when I was interviewing people with diabetes. So many told me diabetes had actually improved their lives. When Saul, a 60-year-old man, was diagnosed with type 2 diabetes, he said, "I'm going to get on top of this." He found a bicycle in his father-in-law's attic and began riding. Since then, he's lost 100 pounds (45.4 kg) and rides 90 miles (145 km) a week. One group he rides with mentors troubled teens and he says this feeds his soul.

Nicole Johnson, a former Miss America, got type 1 diabetes shortly before the pageant. They wanted her to drop out, but she walked down that runway with her insulin pump and all and has gone on to work in public health as a role model for millions.

She says, "I have experienced the power of holding a flourishing mindset. It's what pushes me out the door every morning to walk for an hour, rewards me with good feelings when I eat healthy food, and has me check my blood sugar frequently and correct it in real time. Seeing the better health my actions bring me, and patting myself on the back for my efforts, gives me enormous pleasure and pride."

If you experience thoughts like these:
- *I am terrible at counting carbohydrates.*
- *Nothing I do works.*
- *How in the world am I going to lose 20 pounds (9 kg)?*

Try answering them from a flourishing mindset:
- I am terrible at counting carbohydrates. *This is hard, but when I think about it, I've learned new things before by applying myself and not giving up. I'll get a book tomorrow on carb counting and start with breakfast. I can do this. (See strengths that you already have.)*

- Nothing I do works. *Boy, I'm hard on myself. I do many things that work like taking my walk now after lunch. I feel really good about that. (Recognize your accomplishments and have pride.)*

- How in the world am I going to lose 20 pounds (9 kg)? *Well, if I lost the weight I could enjoy my grandchildren more. I'll call my doctor tomorrow and get a referral to a dietitian. (See what you want and move toward it.)*

I tell people I'm healthier than I would have been without diabetes and that you can have a great life, not despite, but because of diabetes. Each day, look at one thing you're doing well with your diabetes, aim toward where you want to go, and appreciate your efforts. That's a flourishing mindset.

Feel and Share Your Emotions

Many people are uncomfortable sharing deeply personal emotions. Others may feel that they need to be strong for their loved ones and put on a cheerful face. Either way, there are major downsides to holding your emotions inside.

In one twelve-year study, people who reported they preferred to suppress emotions had a 70 percent higher risk of developing cancer and a 47 percent higher risk of developing heart disease.[46] We do not know the causal relationship, but a wide variety of psychological research points to the power of voicing emotions to improve your emotional wellbeing and the physical wellbeing that follows.

You can share emotions privately through a journal, socially through a trusted friend, or professionally through a licensed therapist. The important thing is that you put words to your emotions and face them rather than ignoring them. As a therapist urged his patient, "go through emotions, not around them. You must feel an emotion, sometimes deeply, in order to move beyond it."

Avoid Negative Coping Strategies

Sometimes, we try and flee from our negative emotions. We bury them with drugs, food, shopping, or other things that don't really help us move forward. Some negative coping strategies include the following:

- Drugs, including alcohol and cigarettes
- Eating, either binging or purging
- Withdrawing from social situations
- Emotional outbursts
- Impulse shopping
- Procrastination
- Denial, pretending that nothing's wrong

To correct a negative coping strategy, you need to identify which ones you are using. Are you overeating when frustrated? Are you procrastinating treating your blood sugars? Are you in a state of denial and ignoring diabetes altogether? Once you are consciously aware of the negative coping strategy, you can start to chart a path forward.

You can choose from a wide variety of positive coping strategies to replace your negative ones, such as the following:

- Reframing, changing your internal dialogues
- Expressing your emotions
- Hobbies, expressing yourself creatively
- Working, taking on a new project, or volunteering
- Socializing, surrounding yourself with people who make you feel better
- Setting goals, creating a plan for the future and making progress towards it
- Managing time well, focusing on alleviating things that are causing stress in your life
- Exercising, walking, or dancing your way to better health

- Caring for yourself, focusing on your basic needs
- Caring for your environment, making the spaces around you conducive to your lifestyle goals
- Faith, praying or meditating about the things that give your life meaning
- Relaxing, through movement, a long bath, or meditation

What works will be very specific to you. Speaking with someone else, such as a licensed therapist, can be a productive way to get an outside perspective, identify your unproductive habits, and create a plan to change them.

Mental Health Issues

Many people with diabetes expect their physician to help them with emotional challenges. They become angry or frustrated when the physician goes right past those concerns to address other medical needs on his checklist. The examining room encounter is not meant to be the central place for addressing these important issues. You can mention them, certainly, but do not be surprised if he or she wants you to get these services elsewhere. That is typically in your best interest.

If you feel that your doctor is not responsive to the emotional issues you're dealing with, it simply may be that his or her training was different than the professional who trained to explore emotional issues. He or she may feel that their responsibility is in a different domain and that you will be better served going elsewhere for this type of guidance. Ask your doctor about his preference or comfort level in your bringing emotional issues into the examination room.

It is not enough to acknowledge the difference in expectations of the exam room encounter. There must be a plan that allows you to manage emotional aspects of your life with diabetes. You may have to make it happen on your own, but you should feel free to discuss it briefly with your "diabetes doctor" or "diabetes nurse," even if they do not consider it part of the their role in managing your diabetes. They may or may not know where to suggest you go for this other work on your diabetes. You may feel confused about that separation. The separation is common.

What you need is a plan to do both, separately if necessary. Each professional involved in the medical and emotional management of your diabetes should communicate with the others with regard to their findings and recommendations. You should receive a copy of these communications, so you can put it all together in a way that makes sense to you. You can use teach back (page 140) to the greatest advantage when there appears to be different recommendations about what you think is the same issue.[47] You want to close that gap if you believe they are related to one another in some way that the professionals do not understand clearly. It may allow you to reframe a lot of what you think and feel about your diabetes. If you do that, you may be pleasantly surprised at the new energy and focus unleashed by things you have known about for a long time.

PRACTICE MINDFULNESS

Are you having trouble reframing your thoughts around diabetes? Consider complimenting this approach by practicing mindfulness. The Greater Good Science Center at the University of Berkeley introduces mindfulness this way:

> *Mindfulness means maintaining a moment-by-moment awareness of our thoughts, feelings, bodily sensations, and surrounding environment. Mindfulness also involves acceptance, meaning that we pay attention to our thoughts and feelings without judging them—without believing, for instance, that there's a "right" or "wrong" way to think or feel in a given moment. When we practice mindfulness, our thoughts tune into what we're sensing in the present moment rather than rehashing the past or imagining the future.*

The idea of slowing down and observing the world without judgment may seem like a silly concept to you. How can sitting still possibly improve your wellbeing? In fact, there is a body of research that shows that practicing mindfulness can be as effective as Cognitive Behavioral Therapy.[49] In some studies, those with recurring depression cut their risk of future episodes in half. That's a lot of power for something as simple as slowing down enough to pay attention! Practicing mindfulness is a straightforward process:

1. **Find a quiet, comfortable space.** You want to be in natural light or keep the lights on so that you don't get sleepy.

2. **Sit comfortably in a chair or on the ground.** You have seen pictures of people meditating. Don't feel pressure to adopt a specific position. You just want to have good posture and feel comfortable.

3. **Listen to your breath.** Now it is time to slowly observe your breathing. Listen to the sound of the air going steadily in and out. Your mind will naturally start to wander. When you notice your mind is wandering, return it gently back to your breathing. Do not judge your thoughts. Acknowledge them and return to your breath.

This is a very simple but powerful process. It activates a different way of thinking, focusing you on the direct experience of the immediate moment.[50]

It turns out that when you think about the future, you tend to ignore the present. But when you focus on the present, it relieves you of concerns about the future. The simple act of gaining awareness of your present moment helps release you from your existing habits of thinking and feeling.

If you need help practicing mindfulness, you can reach out to a mental health professional or find resources online or at your local bookstore.

A Pencil Can Make You Happy

Perhaps you have more control over your happiness than you know. In *Thinking, Fast and Slow*, Nobel Prize-winner Daniel Kahneman shares the story of the surprising power of a pencil to influence your mood. If you put a pencil across your mouth and look in the mirror, you naturally smile. Then, surprisingly, you actually feel happier, too. On the other hand, if you put the eraser in your mouth, then you frown. And your emotions follow.

We have remarkable power over our own habits. Something as simple as faking a smile can improve your mood. So develop the habit of finding your own little reasons for gratitude. Find the silver lining in the clouds around you. It's a first step, but a big one. You always have the pencil, and probably a lot more, to get you smiling.

Your emotions are critically important to your success in managing diabetes. Don't let them manage you. You need to manage them. Not so simple? Perhaps. Don't try to make it perfect. Try to make it good enough to get started. And do just that: get started.

Chapter 11

Banish Burnout and Diabetes Distress

Some studies say that as many as 35 percent of people with diabetes are depressed. But this is not accurate. Dealing with diabetes can cause many of the symptoms of depression without adding up to actual clinical depression. It's easy to understand how this happens. You are getting frustrated at pricking your finger at every meal. You can't sleep at night because you're worried about your future. You feel like no one around you has a clue about what you're going through.

Sam was not looking forward to lunch, as he rarely did these days. His office was located right next to Paolo's Pasta Buffet. Again, his co-workers had voted to go there for a fast and inexpensive meal.

Sam had grown up loving pasta. He had always requested spaghetti with homemade meatballs as his birthday dinner. Nothing made him happier. Then he was diagnosed with diabetes.

As he wandered in the doors of the Paolo's Pasta Buffet for the fiftieth time since he was diagnosed, he would yet again have to settle for their despised salad bar. He felt increasingly bitter about it, especially with all of his friends bringing back plates piled high with pasta. Sam didn't know if he could go on with this for the rest of his life.

Who wouldn't feel distressed in this situation—or when your doctor says you have complications?

> *Time slowed to a stop for Tara as she heard the words. "You have peripheral neuropathy."*
>
> *Of all the complications of diabetes, damage to her nerves was the one that scared her the most. She knew the damage was often irreversible. She had seen the effects first hand and shuddered to think of it happening to her.*
>
> *Tara imagined how the pain would grow and slowly creep up from her feet. Even worse, she dreaded when she wouldn't be able to feel the pain at all. What little cut would she miss? What would happen if she got an infection and didn't notice in time?*
>
> *Tara saw her doctor's lips moving, but she hadn't a clue what he was saying. She couldn't make her brain think.*

HALLMARKS OF DIABETES DISTRESS

The appearance of complications can easily cause distress and lead to symptoms of depression. You start by breaking plans or withdrawing socially. You sleep too much or way too little. You feel irritable and lose interest in things you used to care about. Your thoughts slow down. You may start to think that it's not worth it to go through all this.

In recent years, these thoughts and feelings have been called diabetes distress. In moderation, these feelings are normal. In extreme cases, however, it can add up to a clinical depression that needs to be treated. A survey by William Polonsky, Ph.D., founder of the Behavioral Diabetes Institute, available at www.dthrive.com/distress, can help you identify whether you are experiencing diabetes distress and how severe it is. Here are some of the questions the survey asks you to rate on a six-point scale, ranging from "not a problem" to "a very serious problem".[51]

Are you:

- Feeling overwhelmed by the demands of living with diabetes?
- Feeling angry, scared, and/or depressed when you think about living with diabetes?
- Feeling like you're failing with your diabetes depression?
- Feeling that diabetes controls your life?
- Feeling that friends or family do not appreciate how difficult living with diabetes can be?
- Feeling that your doctor doesn't take your concerns seriously enough?

It is challenging to come up with one-sized-fits-all solutions for issues with diabetes distress. Everyone has different ways of thinking about how diabetes impacts the different parts of their life. Once you identify the specific things causing distress, you can start to craft specific solutions. You may work with your support network, which we will talk about in depth in Chapter 12, to solve the problems causing you distress and help you change your behavior, while reframing your feelings and thoughts, in ways that work for you.

For example, if you are feeling overwhelmed by diabetes, you will want to look for ways to reduce the daily burden of diabetes management. Remember: you don't need to do everything at once. And you don't have to be perfect. Take your time.

Speak with a Therapist

It can be challenging to process strong emotions like anger and fear. These are reasonable responses to diabetes. If the source of all these feelings goes beyond the practical aspects of managing diabetes, it may be worthwhile to speak with a licensed therapist. Talk therapy has shown to be very effective in helping people change the way they think about stressful feelings and tasks like managing diabetes.

Speaking with someone is not a sign of personal weakness or failure. Getting an outside perspective on living with diabetes can help you see your own patterns of thought and how to work to reframe unhealthy ones. A professional can help you identify your triggers before they send you careening down an awful emotional highway. Once you understand how and why you are thinking a certain way, you have a much greater ability to change your feelings, thoughts, and behaviors.

One of the side effects of diabetes distress is slowing down your thinking. Reducing the amount of distress that you are experiencing can make other aspects of diabetes significantly easier to manage.

The efforts you make are worth it. Studies show that a combined effort to manage both the emotional side of diabetes stress and the logistics of diabetes management is extremely effective and improves your sense of wellbeing.[50, 51]

Diabetes distress does not belong in the examination room with your diabetes doctor or nurse. It is a related issue with very different demands, different solutions, and different ways of measuring success.

DISTRESS LEADS TO BURNOUT

Over time, feelings of distress can build, leading to a period of burnout. You get fed up with dealing with diabetes and check out. Short periods of burnout are common and may not be something to worry about. However, if you are burned out and check out of your diabetes self-care for an extended period, it can lead to negative consequences for your wellbeing.

We've found two excellent books that can walk you through managing diabetes burnout. The first is *Diabetes Burnout* by Bill Polonsky. The second is *Dealing with Diabetes Burnout* by Ginger Vieira. You can get more information on both books at www.dthrive.com/burnout. Both books begin by acknowledging how common and normal diabetes burnout is. It is no surprise that working a 24-hour-a-day job can leave one feeling exhausted by it! Each person has a different reason for their diabetes burnout. The causes are as varied as the people experiencing it.

But what to do about it? The books walk you through strategies for solving some of the common causes of diabetes burnout. For example, are you seeking perfection rather than accepting "good enough?" Are your expectations for managing diabetes unrealistic? Are you investing a lot of energy into things that aren't helping? If you are experiencing diabetes burnout, we highly recommend diving into one of these guides on the subject. It is absolutely worth it to help manage some of the challenging emotional issues that can arise around diabetes.

It is also important to bring up diabetes burnout with your doctor. Diabetes burnout can put you in a dangerous position where you are not taking adequate care of your blood sugars and putting yourself in harm's way. Your doctor can be an ally in helping you separate the process of managing your blood sugars from your need to overcome burnout. When experiencing burnout, extra support can be especially useful.

Be cautious if your health care professional suggests that getting your blood sugars stabilized will get rid of the diabetes burnout. Frequently, the cause of burnout is not practical, but emotional. So solving the practical problem of daily management won't necessarily solve the emotional one. This is why it's especially important to find the root cause of your burnout so you can focus your efforts on solving the correct problem. That said, having blood sugars that are frequently too high or too low can make burnout worse. It doesn't feel very good and makes diabetes much more burdensome to manage.

ARE YOU DEPRESSED?

There is no easy dividing line between diabetes distress or burnout and clinical depression. It is ultimately determined by the impact it has on your life. If your feelings of distress linger and fester, then it is important to seek help.

One of the great challenges of depression is that when you need help most, you can feel like you might never be able to get out of bed again. You may start to feel like a failure, like you don't deserve to get help, that these feelings are inevitable. You may feel like there's no way out. Sometimes, people feel like they shouldn't be depressed.

Depression doesn't always strike when things are going poorly. You can be rich, happy, and on your way to a new life. You can feel good about your health. There can be no obvious signs of things going wrong. Depression can happen to anyone at any time.

Sometimes depression is triggered by a hormonal change, like having a baby, stopping breastfeeding, or undergoing menopause. Men also have hormonal triggers for depression. Signs of these include loss of muscle strength, decreased physical endurance, sexual dysfunction with erectile failure, and a decreased sex drive. Sometimes it's directly related to the relentless demands of managing diabetes. Other times it seems to have no recognizable cause at all.

Author Allie Brosh has a famous comic about her experience with depression. You can read this comic at www.dthrive.com/depressioncomic and www.dthrive.com/depressioncomic2. Allie shares how her sadness came out of nowhere, consumed her, and left her empty. She eventually tries to get angry at herself, but finds that she doesn't even feel those emotions anymore. She would be in a situation where she was supposed to feel sadness and would struggle to put on her sad face when she felt so lifeless. This experience will ring true to anyone who has walked in her shoes.

After Michelle had a baby, when she felt she should have been happiest, depression struck. She had the baby blues.

Baby Blues

"I just can't do this right now!" Michelle said, tears rolling down her cheeks. Michelle's HbA1c had risen to about 8% for the first time in five years. She was frustrated that nothing seemed to be working. She was doing the best she could, and it just wasn't good enough anymore.

Her doctor turned to her. Pointing to her heart, he said, "Take care of this first, and the diabetes will take care of itself."

She took a deep breath. "I'll try."

Soon after, Michelle started taking an antidepressant and seeing a therapist every week. It was slow going, but over the course of a year, her feelings of depression faded and she felt more like her old self again. And like her doctor promised, her HbA1c started drifting back to where it was before the depression.

Balanced Body and Mind

Michelle's experience is all too common. Luckily, she had a doctor who facilitated her processing her depression and worked with her closely during this period.

Dealing with depression and diabetes requires a balanced approach. We mean this literally: you must find a balance between your body and your mind. As you heal your body, you may find that your mind starts to heal. Or as you heal your mind, you may find that your body starts to heal.

One of the first things you can do is ease up on expectations. Rather than seeking perfection, seek balance. This can help release some of the pressure you put on yourself. As Michelle discovered, taking care of your mind can heal your body. As a confounder, depression can make a low A1c unachievable. That's okay. You need to come first.

On the flip side, if you're depressed because of the diabetes itself, major blood sugar swings can start a negative cycle. You get angry at your diabetes, your diabetes makes you feel bad, and this reinforces your anger. So you must seek balance. This requires a combination of approaches.

First, you may need extra support managing your diabetes during this period. Reading this book is a great step in that direction. It might also help to explain your situation to your doctor or nurse and check in more frequently.

Second, you may join the millions who have had success treating mild to moderate depression with psychotherapy. Working with a licensed social worker (LSW) therapist, psychologist, or psychiatrist, you can begin to understand and change your thought patterns. You can recognize the triggers that cause those patterns and give yourself an opportunity to manage your feelings. Having an outside perspective can help you understand ways of thinking that are so ingrained, you no longer notice them. This gives you the ability to direct your thoughts in a more productive direction.

Third, you may be prescribed an antidepressant medication. Medication has helped many people, though it is often an imperfect solution. You may need to try multiple medications before you find one that works for you. And antidepressants can take more than a month to start working. Many medications must also be stopped slowly or they can cause dangerous side effects.

Ironically, antidepressants can make you feel empty, inhibit your sex drive, or otherwise mute your emotions in order to work. Some of them can also increase blood sugar levels. If you are taking medication to manage depression, ask your prescribing physician or pharmacist about whether it increases blood sugars. Some medications can make blood sugars harder to manage right at the time when you are having the most trouble. Others can have an indirect impact by disrupting sleep.

Lastly, exercise can be an extremely useful approach. In a number of studies, exercise has been shown to be more effective than medication at treating mild to moderate depression, often with longer-lasting effects.

Ask yourself: if your diabetes went away tomorrow, would you still be depressed? This can help you focus on where to start. Depression can be an enormous burden to carry alone. If you feel you are depressed, gather your personal strength and reach for help. Call your doctor, explain that you are feeling depressed, and get a referral to someone that can help you create a plan. You've gotten to the end of this book, a clear sign that you want to take charge of your own health. Don't delay now.

You may feel like depression is your fault. You may feel like you are weak because you can't snap out of it. This is not the case. Depression is very common, but it is not a normal state of living. It often requires help from someone else to get through to the other side.

Chapter 12

Build Your Support Network

Thriving is not something you often do on your own. We are all social beings. We look for connections, to be part of a greater community. We often want or need help when we stumble. Diabetes can work against this natural tendency. It can be isolating. In some cases, it can hurt relationships.

Thriving with diabetes requires a healthy social environment around you. Sometimes, this means minimizing the impact of a negative influence, like a co-worker who complains about your too-healthy diet. It can also be very positive, like finding a peer with diabetes who understands you and with whom you can share problem-solving efforts without judgment.

If you are going to thrive with diabetes, you need to be selective about who you allow to be part of your support team and the role that they should play. In this section, we will look at how you manage diabetes in the various relationships in your life and suggest new kinds of relationships that will help you not just live with diabetes, but thrive.

YOUR MEDICAL TEAM

When you envision your diabetes support team, you probably think first about your doctor. This makes sense, since your doctor prescribes your medication and explains how to use it. However, the medical team is not equipped to be a support team.

You can help your doctor be more effective in the support role by using the "teach back" method we discussed earlier. By repeating your doctor's suggestions to ensure you are in agreement, you can prevent many of the missteps that so often happen. Instructions that seem clear to the doctor often have a way of getting muddied in your mind by the time you get home. Because teach back is so effective, the American Board of Internal Medicine recommends this method and trains doctors to use it effectively. But don't wait for them—you can start the teach back so you know that the doctor said what he meant to say and you heard it the way he intended. Just say, "I want to share with you what I just heard to make sure I have it right." That usually works if the doctor wants to be clear. Then the doctor is more likely to speak with you and not "at you."

This can help improve how your doctor supports you. Maybe your teach back shows him that your situation has changed in ways he didn't recognize before. Sharing your version of the information may change the recommendations he or she makes for your treatment. This makes you a key member of the medical team for your diabetes care, as you should be.

As Sarah discovered, speaking up during a doctor visit can transform the whole outcome.

Just Say It!

Sarah's doctor was halfway out of the room when she said, "There's one more thing." He turned back and she continued. "This may sound strange, but my handwriting in the afternoon feels weird. I don't know how else to describe it."

"Has anything else changed?" her doctor asked.

"Well, I don't know. I've been trying to lose weight by cutting down my carbs at lunch. But how would that be connected?"

"Have you adjusted your insulin since our last visit?"

Sarah's doctor guessed very quickly that she was experiencing mild low blood sugars in the early afternoon. Sarah hadn't noticed because they tended to be back up above her target range by dinner.

Sarah's doctor adjusted her afternoon insulin and asked her to check her blood sugar in the mid-afternoon and before dinner over the next few days and call him back in three days to confirm it was working.

Sarah called back the next week to report that she was feeling better, her handwriting was back to normal, and she was pleasantly surprised to find that her blood sugars were consistently where she wanted them to be before dinner.

FAMILY, FRIENDS, AND CO-WORKERS

Improving your communication with your doctor is critical. But who is going to help you during the 8,756 hours you are not with your doctor each year? Who will help with all the day-to-day decision-making you need to do? So many of your decisions about what you eat, when you exercise, and how you manage the emotional ups and downs of diabetes are influenced by the people around you.

The key skill for creating a positive social environment for managing diabetes is negotiation. Think about how the people in your life can best support you. This means getting clear about what you want them to do and what you don't want them to do. With a partner, it can mean setting some ground rules for communication. For example:

- Please do not comment on my dessert choices. Sometimes, I don't want to be reminded of my diabetes. Sometimes, I need a break. To help, maybe you could pick up berries and whipped cream on the next trip to the grocery? There are fewer carbohydrates in that than the ice cream, and I could still get my fix. But if I choose to have ice cream, please don't comment.

- When I'm low, please bring me a juice box but don't talk to me. I like to sit quietly until I feel better. When you try to engage me, I feel frustrated and exhausted. Sometimes, I just need a little space to get back to myself.

- If we are having an argument and you say, "you're just grumpy because you have high blood sugar," this makes me feel like you are discounting my opinion. Instead, please say that you think I may have high blood sugar and let's take care of that and then finish the discussion.

Sometimes, family and friends can be supportive, but it can be a challenge for even the best-intentioned family supporters to help. A caring but critical remark can feel judgmental.

Setting Boundaries

Sara was going to go to her grandma's house in Chicago for the holidays, but decided she would skip it this year. Last year, as she went for seconds of cranberry sauce, her aunt said loudly, "Sara, should you really be eating that?" Soon all sixteen people around the table were debating Sara's food habits and what she was doing to herself.

"So this year I'm going to skip it," Sara said to her doctor with tears in her eyes.

Her doctor responded that Sara's aunt may not realize how much that comment embarrassed her and would regret the comment. Sara agreed, but didn't know how to handle it. Her doctor suggested that she go to her grandma's house, give her aunt a big hug, ask to speak with her privately, and say, "I almost didn't come this year. My diabetes is very private to me and I do not like to discuss it publicly. It's as private to me as it would be talking about you going to the bathroom at the dinner table."

So, Sara went to her Grandma's house. Her aunt was shocked when they spoke. She had no idea that Sara had felt that way and felt guilty about it. She apologized profusely. Sara had a great time with her family.

Write Your Own Script

People ask questions like, "should you be eating that?" for a lot of reasons. They might be concerned about your health. They could be nosy or malicious. Either way, this is a place for you to set clear boundaries. You might respond with your own question: "Honestly, that's a personal topic that I would prefer not to discuss. How would it feel if someone walked around questioning each of your food choices?"

There are times when you should make sure that someone in your social group knows you have diabetes, can interpret signs you are having a problem, and support you. This is especially true if you are doing something potentially dangerous like hiking, sailing, or even playing golf. It isn't something that you should feel obligated to share with everyone. Instead, we recommend confiding in someone that you trust, for your own safety.

When doing any activities that involve food, it can be useful to broadcast your food preferences rather than being private about them. This can be as simple as, "what menu are you planning? I am eating a lower carbohydrate diet, and it would really help to have some low-carb options. I'm happy to bring something to share if it would help." Most people are happy to make accommodations.

The truth is, people without diabetes often don't understand it as well as they think they might. Many, and possibly most, of the frustrating and hurtful comments that you hear are due to a misunderstanding, rather than malice. Spending a few moments to think about who needs to know, and doing a little education with that person, can go a long way towards building a successful support team.

Choose a Trusted Colleague

Remember Jack, who experienced unpredictable low blood sugars on the afternoons when he ran around the factory servicing machines? He had a lot of success by making his co-worker aware of the symptoms of his low blood sugars and what that person could do to help when he became low. A trusted colleague can be an integral part of your support network at work.

You may want to fortify that relationship by inviting another co-worker to act in a similar role. It is important to be explicit about how someone can help you and make sure they are comfortable doing so. It could be as simple as, "Hey, John, if I say 'I'm low' or you think I might be, could you grab me a juice box from my desk drawer?"

It is important to be selective about whom you reach out to for this type of support, especially at work. To some, this may feel like an unwanted obligation. Telling your boss about your needs at work is more straightforward than asking a colleague for help.

Sometimes, you don't have a choice about the people that you work, live, or play with. The challenges of negotiating how they interact around your diabetes can be as hard as any other deeply emotional, high-stakes conversation about love or finances.

If you are having trouble talking with others about your diabetes, we recommend a book like *Crucial Conversations* or *Difficult Conversations*. Both of these step-by-step guides can you help navigate boundaries and ask for help from a spouse, friend, co-worker, or boss.

PEER MENTORS AND GROUPS[54]

Other people who are living with diabetes can play a uniquely positive role in your life. A peer's understanding of what you're going through can help you think through the many intimate and practical decisions you need to make all the time. They can also help you achieve your potential to thrive.

This makes a lot of sense when you think about other parts of your life. Discussing difficult decisions around relationships or finances with someone who has gone through similar experiences can be both clarifying and comforting. Those who truly understand us can be our biggest supporters. Very often, peer mentors are groups of two. But when people form larger groups, it can be transformative for the participants. The Youngstown Pump Club was one such place where a wide variety or participants came together to succeed. The group learned together about how to handle different situations. If someone's blood sugars were getting high, they would go down the list of confounders or suggest changes to the pump site or type of insulin. Some people came frequently, others less often. Everyone had a different reason to be there. But everyone listened and worked together on the various problems that arose. And it worked. Participants thrived.

Increased Brainpower and Empathy

A peer mentor group, whether it's you and a friend or an organized one like the Youngstown Pump Club, provides two benefits. On one hand, you get all the brainpower in your group applied to solving your problems. But it's more than that—you also get a chance to help solve the problems of others. As the needs of different members of the group change, so do the conversations. The goal isn't always to find the perfect answer, but to help each person in the room think through their options and find a path works for them. There's growing research on the social dynamics and decision-making processes that make these groups succeed:[52]

No One Is "In Charge"

First, to be effective, peer groups have to be careful about the relationship between the participants and the group. Each person must understand the limitations of the group. There are often gaps in the information that you share or receive. It can be impractical, incomplete, incorrect, or unsafe.

In recognition that each person is taking charge of their own care, these groups are best without a formal leader. This does not mean there can be no administrative leader who organizes the sessions. And people can take turns facilitating the discussion, ensuring that each person has an opportunity to share their perspective. However, one person shouldn't be in the position of deciding whose opinion, experience, or information matters and whose does not. As a peer group, it is for people to determine by themselves and for the group to decide together in consensus. However, it is important to make sure that you don't outsource your decision-making to the group even when there is consensus. You are in charge of your self-care, so make sure you agree with something before acting on it.

What's Not on the Table: Meds

Second, groups must carefully determine what types of discussions are appropriate and which ones are not. Peers should not be guiding you in how to take medication. That's the role of your doctor. However, they may suggest strategies that you can discuss with your doctor. Moreover, your peers can help you in ways that your doctor can't. This is especially true when it comes to changing your habits.

In the Youngstown Pump Club, the founder cultivated awareness of these boundaries. An insulin pumper who had diabetes for over twenty years, she was careful not to allow people in the group to make medication adjustment recommendations or specific insulin pump adjustments to other people in the group, without that person consulting their physician. It was about how one approached their own self-care success, not calculating a dose of insulin.

As we discuss throughout this book, diabetes is about so much more than how much insulin or medication to take. Instead, a peer group focuses on a wide range of diabetes experiences. Often, the Youngstown group invited doctors and nurses to join sessions. When a new insulin pump was released, they would be dissecting the new features with the help of a representative from the insulin pump company. Additionally, the people in the group reached out to each other outside the meetings, and to their physicians, as well as nurses, dietitians, pharmacists, and educators to confirm information discussed at meetings. They brought the information assessment back to the group for further conversation, clarification, and adjustment of the consensus. The insulin pump became a common and compelling bond that has helped to sustain this group for over 25 years.

Repetition Reinforces Group Knowledge

Third, groups should value the experience that each person brings. One of the great benefits to a group like this is what author and consultant Kate Pugh calls "hidden know how".[53] This is the unique collection of thoughts and experiences that each person brings to a discussion. She likens it to a jazz performance, where people come together and create something new and special that would be impossible for one to create on their own. Each person is speaking in their own voice and then it comes together in an "aha! moment." When people drift in and out of meetings, it becomes a hidden advantage. If they weren't there to hear what happened at an earlier meeting, a review of the information often reframes the conversation in important ways to reflect an unexamined angle. It makes everyone in the room smarter.

Peer Accountability

The benefits that flow from a good peer group are tremendous. You can trust the first-hand knowledge of your peers in a way that you might not trust it coming from a well-meaning expert.

Moreover, in addition to all of that knowledge, you get the ongoing support in changing your habits and sustaining those changes that we discussed in Chapter 11. Changing your own behavior is one of the greatest challenges of managing diabetes. This is especially true if you've been eating a certain way your whole life or are adopting an exercise program for the first time. Lifelong habits are particularly stubborn.

Peer mentors not only provide insight into how to problem solve around your diabetes, but can also hold you accountable in ways that others can't. They get it. They are dealing with the same issues. So when you both agree to make a change, it's much easier to hold each other to it.[53]

Peer Support Online

Over the last fifteen years, the internet has made it possible to easily connect with peer mentors. These communities include the following:

- Diabetes Daily (www.diabetesdaily.com)
- TuDiabetes (www.tudiabetes.org)
- EsTuDiabetes (www.estudiabetes.org) in Spanish
- Children with Diabetes (www.childrenwithdiabetes.com)
- Search Facebook for Pages and Groups about diabetes.
- See an expanded list at www.dthrive.com/peersupport.

PUT YOURSELF FIRST

This book is about more than helping you succeed. That comes first, but over time, we also hope to contribute to a change in the way our health care system treats people with diabetes.

There has been a vibrant conversation in recent years about how our health care system is actually a sick care system. It is not designed to maintain health but treat sickness. Diabetes and other chronic conditions are not well supported. Sometimes, they make you acutely sick, but most often it is a chronic challenge.

This must change. It is in all of our best interests to have a health system that can support people living with chronic conditions like diabetes. Research confirms what we all know intuitively: early investments in helping you find a sustainable way to manage diabetes will improve your health decades from now. The savings in both dollars and suffering are real.

Unfortunately, the financial savings don't kick in during the first twelve months. Plus, effective programs tend to be more time-consuming and hard to automate using technology. They require more personal engagement, investigation, and ongoing interactions. They don't start and stop, like surgery. The effectiveness of programs for chronic illness are difficult to measure because the payoff may be years in the future. Further, measuring "success" or health benefits are easier if you focus on medical procedures that make money for those who provide them than it is to measure benefit from expensive services that help you achieve lifelong health. There have been few incentives for organizations to invest in programs that create sustainable outcomes because it is so difficult to monitor processes and measure both financial and practical benefits of sustainability over time.

Health care reform efforts are slowly changing this. There is a movement towards paying doctors not based on the number of procedures they perform—an enormous incentive to give you as many tests and surgeries as possible—but based on measures that reflect sustaining your health in the presence of chronic disorders like diabetes. If a doctor can help you achieve better health than average, they can make more money. If they are less successful, they make less. Why would they spend money on procedures and tests that don't work very well when they could empower people with diabetes to take charge of their own health?

Thankfully, you don't need to wait for the health care system to change. Using the tools in this book, you can stand up for your needs and make sure the system meets them. It's not always easy, but we believe that you have the ability to do it.

HELP OTHERS TOUCHED BY DIABETES

Would you like to help others thrive with diabetes? There are many ways to get involved, from educating your doctor about your needs, to joining a peer mentor group, to pushing insurance companies when they deny coverage, to voting for legislators who understand your needs.

In your one-on-one interactions, you can take the time to share your experience. Correct misconceptions about diabetes. We know how frustrating those can be, but they are so often out of ignorance and rarely out of spite.

If an insurance company denies a request for reimbursement, appeal that response. Insurance companies often say no until they feel like patient demand is genuinely high. For example, coverage for continuous glucose meters has dramatically expanded over the last few years in part due to the passionate letters written by people living with diabetes and their doctors. Too many insurance companies have a policy of "just say no" until someone pushes back. So push back!

It is also important for people with diabetes to have political power. When we speak with political representatives, they explain that no one ever calls them to talk about diabetes as an issue. This needs to change. So if you see an issue that you care about, take a moment to call or send an email. It's even better to set up an appointment in your local office. If you want to see bills impacting people with diabetes and steps that you can take to help, then visit www.dthrive.com/advocate.

This book is just the beginning of the conversation. We are committed to helping you, and everyone else living with diabetes, to thrive. To continue your journey, you can find more support at the site of our book, www.dthrive.com.

Resources

APPENDIX A: LETTER TO YOUR HEALTH CARE PROVIDER

Dear Health Care Provider,

We wrote this book for patients. However, the processes that we suggest have been used with success in clinical environments. If you find these approaches confluent with your professional judgment, then we invite you to consider them for you own use. Like you, we believe in personalized, evidence-based treatment approaches that consistently deliver positive, verifiable results.

The Process

Thriving with Diabetes is built around a patient-centered action plan that pulls together all we know about managing blood sugar trends prospectively, reducing the cognitive burden of diabetes management, and facilitating an effective doctor/patient relationship. In practice, this program has been confluent with a wide range of existing approaches to diabetes clinical care.

The 4-step action plan is laid out in Part Two of the book:

Step 1: Lower the Highs. Diabetes is first and foremost a condition of high blood sugar. This process focuses on the tools necessary to lower high blood sugars.

Step 2: Limit the Lows. Once you begin lowering high blood sugars, the patient inevitably experiences low blood sugars. This chapter shows people how to identify, prevent, and treat hypoglycemia.

Step 3: Use Your Best to Fix the Rest. This is an iterative and self-reinforcing patient-driven educational process. Unlike most other diabetes management approaches, this allows patients to anticipate glucose trends that approach target values and correct those that don't. This prospective process is better than a retrospective one that is focused on mitigating negative events that have already happened and cannot be undone.

Step 4: Play with Your Diabetes. This process teaches the patient to navigate changes that cause a breakdown in the predictability of their blood sugars. An extension of the previous step, it is an iterative approach to problem-solving while erring on the side of safety to avoid hypoglycemia. These life changes can be anything from a simple time change to a new child to a catastrophic illness. This chapter focuses on developing the patient's skills for sustainable self-care—with safety and optimism.

Together, the full *Thriving with Diabetes* process responds to a very uncomfortable truth. We all know that diabetes is a serious disease. But it is one thing to say this and another to watch young people implode from complications and die awful deaths. We health care providers give the best care that we can, but we often don't have the time or resources to solve the problems our patients are facing. By the time we can get the resources, diabetes has often progressed too far to undo the damage. Sometimes, aggressive interventions can lead to partial recoveries and mitigation of symptoms. Yet all too often, these efforts exhaust patients emotionally, physically, and financially.

This also leads us to nihilism. We find ourselves physically and emotionally drained. Our efforts are called into question by insurance companies, hospital administrators, and sometimes the patients themselves. However, in spite of these challenges, we know the joys of success. We are driven to help our patients avoid the complications of diabetes and maximize the quality of their lives. We want to succeed for our patients.

Why We Wrote This Book

The journey to create this book began in the early 1990s with a computer model to predict blood sugars. It took into account not just blood sugars and activities, but also the body's hormonal rhythms. Then we encountered a problem: there were so many variables that it choked the computer systems at the time. Diabetes was too complex to model simply.

But we persevered. First, we used the computer model to determine what variables were most impactful on blood sugars and focused on those alone. Second, we looked at shorter time frames. Third, we discovered the existence of "confounders," variables that destroyed the predictive power of the model. For example, chronic pain and sleep disorders made blood sugars hard to predict.

There was a second failure when we worked to transfer from the world of computer-modeling to the real-world demands of a doctor's office. Patients could not collect enough useful information to power the models. Yet again, we had to simplify our models to make them work for patients. This led to the Power of Threes model that we describe in this book. It uses structured checking of blood sugars around blood sugar-impacting events to identify clinically significant and actionable glucose trends. We combined this with education about things that influence blood sugar.

Predicting how blood sugars will change is a key first step to success. The second step—and one where our medical system rarely succeeds—is changing one's behavior. The truth is that physicians are not trained to facilitate behavior change. We are trained to practice medicine. Nurses have a different role and are often trained to teach, but likewise are insufficiently trained in behavior change. This is similarly true for other members of the health care team.

One key to long-term success is empowering patients from the beginning to take charge of self-care behaviors. Patients spend more than 99.9 percent of their time managing diabetes on their own. The way we approach diabetes management must reflect this.

We conclude this book with a variety of strategies for facilitating behavior change. This includes changing one's environment and how one sees it, enhancing motivation, or decreasing the effort required to change a behavior. One of the major benefits of the process in this book is that it simplifies diabetes into smaller, more manageable pieces. This significantly decreases the effort required to make changes.

All of this change is also supported by the patient's social context, something that is not well recognized in the medical environment. The medical environment assumes that the patient is an island unconnected to friends, family, and peers. Yet, these potential supporters of positive change have a major influence on patient behavior.

The clinical focus of diabetes is also unnecessarily negative. Patient successes are swept aside to focus on the parts of diabetes care that are not working. This robs patients of motivation and adds conflict to the doctor/patient relationship. Patients follow the lead of their health care providers by becoming focused on what they are doing wrong and actually discard the things that are working for them.

Lessons for Your Practice

As part of the *Thriving with Diabetes* program, we have identified ways in which the effectiveness of clinical diabetes care can be improved. We urge health care providers to consider the following ideas in their practice of diabetes management:

- We identify confounders early in the book which will hamper the success of anyone with diabetes in creating a maintainable self-care program. We encourage you to evaluate each diabetes patient for these confounders early in the attempt to reach clinical targets. You and your patients will be rewarded with a less burdensome road to reaching those goals and sustaining them if you search for and manage these issues first.

- Physicians should follow a "Use Your Best to Fix the Rest" approach and focus on time periods where patients are successfully managing diabetes rather than those periods when things are not working. You can use these as building blocks for constructing an effective self-management strategy.

The fulcrum of success is identifying when an in-target blood sugar goes out of range and recognizing what caused that to happen.

- The patient should be included as part of the health care team. In the examination room, the doctor is the leader of the interaction and making decisions about the prescription of treatments and the transactions necessary to implement them. Outside of the exam room, the interactions should assume that the patient is leading the self-care efforts and the health care team is in place to support and respond to those efforts.

- Patients should be encouraged to use "teach back" to convey their understanding of the physician's instructions. It is important to make sure that patients are both able and willing to follow them.

- Physicians should emphasize to patients the importance of their social support environment and, recognizing the influence of this environment, interview the patient to gain an understanding of potential areas where social support may be a negative influence. Moreover, physicians should support and, if possible facilitate, the patient developing a relationships with one or more peer mentors.

We support the evolution of recommendations for clinical practice of people with diabetes offered by the American Diabetes Association and American Association of Diabetes Educators. We also applaud the work of the Agency for Health Research and Quality, Medicare Innovation Projects, The Communicable Disease Center Diabetes Translation Division, and others who work to grow diabetes medical care and patient self-management capabilities.

However, gaps remain. Current diabetes education measures are management-based rather than patient-based. The patient-based part of current diabetes management training is, in our judgment, sufficiently haphazard to result in non-sustainable benefits from the early diabetes management teaching currently available.

We believe that diabetes self-care development is a one-year project that leaves patients with achievement goals and a patient-led, multi-focused support system. It creates sustainable, measured, self-care outcomes. Medical care has to be integrated with the support activities that occur in the patients' life. That takes place outside of the examination room, is a measurable process, and can produce measurable results. Changes in the medical team may be needed for adequate diabetes medical and self-care to make this a clinically and economically successful, functional, and consistent component of the health care system.

To succeed, everything outside the examination room has to be patient led. Patients have to be taught to lead in the context of their family, social, and work lives and their diabetes needs. That is thriving with diabetes.

The concepts in this book put together evidence-based approaches in a comprehensive patient-centric system. This is very much a work in progress, and we are grateful for your feedback on how it works in your clinical practice.

Sincerely,
Paul Rosman D.O., F.A.C.P., F.A.C.E.
David Edelman

APPENDIX B: MEDICATIONS THAT LOWER BLOOD SUGAR

This is a list of medications, other than insulin, that lower blood sugars. Most are prescribed for type 2 diabetes, although some are used for type 1 diabetes (even though many are not specifically approved in the United States for use in type 1 diabetes). These medications may be available under a different brand name outside the United States.

MEDICATION FAMILY	HOW IT WORKS	GENERIC NAMES (Brand Names)
Biguanides	· Liver releases less sugar · Muscles use more sugar	**metformin** (Glucophage, Glucophage XR, and Glumetza)
Sulfonylurea	· Pancreas produces more insulin	**glipizide** (Glucotrol), **glimepiride** (Amaryl)
Secretagogue	· Pancreas produces more insulin	**nateglinide** (Starlix), **repaglinide** (Prandin)
Thiazolidinedione	· Muscles use more insulin · Liver releases less sugar	**rosiglitazone** (Avandia), **pioglitazone** (Actos)
Alpha-Glucosidase Inhibitors	· Intestines absorb less sugar	**acarbose** (Precose)
DPP4 inhibitors	· Stimulates glucose-dependent insulin secretion · Decreases glucagon secretion · Slows gastric emptying · Decreases appetite	**sitagliptin** (Januvia), **saxagliptin** (Onglyza), **linagliptin** (Tradjenta), **alogliptin** (Nesina)
Glucagon-like protein 1 receptor agonists (GLP1-RA)	· Stimulates glucose-dependent insulin secretion · Decreases glucagon secretion · Slows gastric emptying · Decreases appetite	**exenatide** (Byetta), **liraglutide** (Victoza), **exenatide extended release** (Bydureon)
Amylin analogues	· Decreases glucagon secretion · Decreases glucagon secretion · Slows gastric emptying · Decreases appetite · Reduces post-meal blood sugars	**pramlintide** (Symlin)
SGLT-2 inhibitors	· Causes you to urinate more glucose	**canagliflozin** (Invokana), **dapagliflozin** (Farxiga), **empagliflozin** (Jardiance)

APPENDIX C: WORKSHEETS

These worksheets are all available for download at www.dthrive.com/worksheets.

Use the Rule of Threes to Predict Your Blood Sugars

You can use this simple process to see how a meal or other activity impacts your blood sugars.

Step 1: Choose a Repetitive Activity

TIME OF DAY	TYPE OF ACTIVITY	DETAILS
Morning Afternoon Evening Night	Meal Physical Activity Emotional/Stressful Event Rest/Napping	Example: oatmeal or yoga class

Step 2: Repeat the Activity on Three Different Days

	DAY 1	DAY 2	DAY 3	
CHECK 1				Check right before activity.
DO THE ACTIVITY				
CHECK 2				MEALS: Check after one hour. OTHER: Check after two hours.
CHECK 3				MEALS: Check before next meal. OTHER: Check after three hours.

Tips for Success

To make events predictable, they must be similar. So start by looking at events that take place on the same kind of days. For example, look at weekdays or weekends separately. If you exercise first thing in the morning, then those days may be different than non-exercise days.

How to Understand the Results

If you consistently get the same change in blood sugar, then that activity is predictable. If your results are inconsistent, return to the four step process. Also, consider the following:

- The events aren't actually the same. Is the content of the meal, level of exertion, time of day, or something else different?

- There is an unrelated activity impacting the results.
    - Are your starting blood sugars vastly different from one another?
    - Was your sleep the same on all 3 nights before the activity occurred?
    - Did you experience a stressful situation?

Sleep Diary

Your sleep patterns have a big impact on your blood sugars.

SLEEP DIARY: STARTING AT NOON ON SUNDAY, SHADE THE AREAS WHEN YOU WERE SLEEPING

	12P	1P	2P	3P	4P	5P	6P	7P	8P	9P	10P	11P	12A	1A	2A	3A	4A	5A	6A	7A	8A	9A	10A	11A
SUN																								
MON																								
TUE																								
WED																								
THU																								
FRI																								
SAT																								
SUN																								
MON																								
TUE																								
WED																								
THU																								
FRI																								
SAT																								

Take a Walk

See how much your blood sugar drops during a short walk. Try this activity when you have not eaten in a few hours or been under stress.

CHECK BLOOD SUGAR:	
TAKE A 20-MINUTE WALK	
CHECK BLOOD SUGAR:	

Did your blood sugars increase? This can be a sign that your body is under stress, such as from physical pain. In some cases, it can be an early warning sign for heart disease. You may want to ask your doctor to perform a stress test if this happens consistently.

Symptom Diary

Use a symptom diary to track the impact of new medications, changed dosages, low blood sugars, or high blood sugars. To use this diary, list any symptoms that you experience across the top, such as a shakiness, numbness, upset stomach, headache, etc. Each day, record how strongly you experience the symptom on a scale of one to five, with five being the strongest.

	Symptom:	Symptom:	Symptom:	Symptom:	Symptom:
Day 1					
Day 2					
Day 3					
Day 4					
Day 5					
Day 6					
Day 7					
Day 8					
Day 9					
Day 10					
Day 11					
Day 12					
Day 13					
Day 14					

Acknowledgments

Many people made this book possible. Some helped support us in deeply personal ways. Others believed in our vision and helped nurture the book along. Many more contributed their ideas and experiences to the world through publicizing their own thinking on a wide variety of topics. We are grateful to them all. We are both especially thankful to our families that supported us through this time-consuming process.

Thank you to Andrea Somberg, our always upbeat and hard-working agent, who helped us frame our ideas, pitch them to publishers, and shepherd the book to completion. If there is a more delightful agent to work with, she must have wings and a halo.

Thank you to Amanda Waddell at Fair Winds Press for betting on our success. Thank you to Renae Haines for managing the publishing process and Laura Smith for her awesome contributions as an editor.

There are also those who helped guide us towards insight and excellence during our careers.

Paul Rosman: I am thankful to my wife, Barbara, and son, Jefferson, for their continuing support through evenings and weekends of working on the book. She gave me the room I needed to press on through many stages of writing and rewriting, while running a busy community-based endocrine practice in Warren, Ohio.

Dr. Scott Pappada did the computer simulations necessary to craft the completed algorithm for glycemic trend prediction in people with diabetes. Brent Cameron facilitated and supported us and took a leadership role in advancing this work at the School of Engineering at the University of Toledo.

Robert Morgan worked with me in bringing the results of earlier studies to a wider audience. I met David Edelman at Bob's urging. It was, and remains, a wonderful gift to be able to work with David. David and I began with presentations at the Diabetes Partnership of Cleveland and then partnered in writing the online course for people with diabetes. Both were foundational in many ways to making this book happen.

As an osteopathic physician, I have always been sensitive to the considerations of primary care physicians because that was the focus of my medical school training. As I ventured into the academic world, I found myself searching for the basic elements of physiology that were both universal and clinically measureable that influenced illness in individuals and could be used to enhance clinical outcomes in individual patients. This book is the product of that work. Drs. Stuart Bondurant and David Goodman at the Albany Medical College gave me a seminal clinical research opportunity which became a vital pillar for this work. Dr. Martin Sonenberg at Memorial Sloan Kettering led me to the world of cell biology and forever changed my views of hormonal processes and their powerful role in individual well-being. At the Downstate Medical Center and Brooklyn Veterans Administration Medical Center, my own clinical research began to move forward in collaboration with Dr. Eleanor Wallace and others and led to a transformative mentorship with chronobiologist Elliott Weitzman.

Yet, all of this failed to answer my original question of how to get science to meet the individual needs of patients. I went into endocrine practice in Warren, Ohio, and within that practice, began to sense an answer among people with diabetes, first, with Scott Pappada in a mutually productive research relationship that has lasted for more than ten years, and ultimately, with David Edelman. Finally, this book captures the answer to my original question of how to apply science to individuals, simply, effectively, and safely and how to achieve our shared purpose. I thank all the people mentioned above and others who are not. Also, the people who David has brought to this effort mentioned below, and I thank David. My family has had a large role in making this book possible and they are uppermost in my thoughts and feelings every day.

I want to acknowledge the people who have entrusted me with their health care over the years and who helped to write this book by their candor, strength, and resourcefulness. They are the people who worked with me in developing diaries that worked. The students, residents, and fellows who provided lessons in relevance. The staff who worked in my office, especially Joan Leonard, and including Debbie, Denise, Colleen, Nancy, and Esther. I was also fortunate to have known Jean Rider, who originated and sustained the Youngstown Pump Club with common sense, excellent judgment, and remarkable expertise.

David Edelman: I am especially grateful for my family's support. My family has a long tradition of working to heal the world, what the Jewish faith calls "tikkun olam." I am grateful to my parents, grandparents, siblings, aunts, uncles and cousins for believing that we can, should, and have an obligation to improve the world for others.

I am thankful to the people with diabetes we name below—as well as so many others who have poured their hearts into the Diabetes Daily community. In particular, I would like to thank Ginger Vieira, who has improved Diabetes Daily through her editorship in countless ways and given me the time I needed to work on this project. I know few people who have worked so hard for the betterment of others and received so little compensation in return."

So many of the ideas in this book were shaped by people living with diabetes and their loved ones. They taught us about the many paths that can lead to success. These include Jessica Apple, Christel Aprigliano, Brandy Barnes, Scott Benner, Marc Bloch, Jeffrey Brewer, Adam Brown, Brian Cohen, Dayton Coles, Emily Coles, Andreina Davila, Larry Dlott, Mike Durbin, Bennet Dunlap, Steven Edelman, Bernard Farrell, Jimmy and Mila Ferrer, Heather Gabel, Bob Geho, Karen Graffeo, Riva Greenberg (and her lovely husband Bou), Manny Hernandez, Donna Hill, Jeff Hitchcock, Mike Hoskins, Scott Johnson, Tom Karlya, Aaron Kowalski, Kelly Kunik, Mike Lawson, Melissa Lee, Leighann Calentine, Laura, Mark, and Jordan Leventhal, Sysy Morales, Ken Moritsugu, Peter Nerothin, Robert Oringer, Bob Pederson, Catherine Price, Kelly Rawlings, Christina Roth, Gary Scheiner, Cherise Shockley, Meri Schuhmacher, Natalie Sera, George Simmons, Phil and Biljana Southerland, Kerri Sparling, Chris Stocker, Lorraine Steihl, David Lee Strasberg, Scott Strange, Scott Strumello, Andreas Stuhr, John Sjolund, Amy Tenderich, Lee Ann Thill, Ginger Vieira, Kim Vlasnik, Bill Woods, and Elizabeth Zabell. There are many, many others who have we are surely forgetting and deserve recognition.

Paul Rosman credits one of his first patients, Jean Rider, whose work with the Youngstown Pump Club gave him an understanding what a peer mentor group could be, even though he didn't know to call it that at the time.

Thank you to the diaTribe team, especially Kelly Close, for investing tens of thousands of hours covering the diabetes industry and sharing their reporting. If you don't get their remarkable free newsletter, sign up at www.diatribe.org. They make us all smarter.

There are hundreds working in the health care system who constantly look for ways to improve how the medical profession approaches diabetes. We have learned a great deal from Bill Polonsky, Hope Warshaw, John Walsh, Ruth Roberts, Adam Kaufman, Anne Peters, Aaron Kowalski, Henry Anhalt, Mark Fendrick, Jen Block, Richard Jackson, Dana Ball, David Panzirer, and John Brooks. Many others are listed in the endnotes.

Thanks also to Rob Muller for investing in the first diabetes social media summit. That face-to-face gathering kicked off a series of collaborations that continue to grow and touch the lives of countless people around the world.

Lastly, thank you to all of those who invest in supporting those living with diabetes. It is a marathon of challenges that few without it can truly understand.

About the Authors

Paul M. Rosman, D.O., F.A.C.P., F.A.C.E., is a clinical endocrinologist committed to helping revolutionize the way diabetes is treated around the world. Trained as a Doctor of Osteopathic Medicine and a Board Certified Internist and Endocrinologist by the American Board of Internal Medicine, he has worked with patients for over 25 years to help them live healthy, happy lives. Dr. Rosman has also lectured throughout the United States and taught at institutions including SUNY Downstate Medical Center in New York, Ohio University, Northern Ohio Medical College, and the University of Toledo Health Science Center in Ohio. He has worked to help advance the field of diabetes in numerous leadership roles. He has chaired chapters of the American Diabetes Association and the American Association of Clinical Endocrinologists and led the medical advisory board of the Ohio Diabetes Prevention and Control Program. He has also served as Senior Medical Advisor to Eli Lilly and Company, the pharmaceutical company that first developed insulin in 1921.

David Edelman is co-founder and CEO of Diabetes Daily, a leading online community for people touched by diabetes. After a loved one was diagnosed with type 1 diabetes, he was driven to create a place where people living with diabetes could connect and work together for a better future. David believes in the power of patient voices to transform not just individual lives, but the entire health system. Through his service to Diabetes Daily, the board of the Diabetes Hands Foundation, and other organizations, he has worked to amplify the voices of those living with diabetes to expand access to quality health care and ensure everyone gets the support they need to succeed.

References

1 Wasserman D. H. & Halseth A. E. An Overview of Muscle Glucose Uptake during Exercise. In Skeletal Muscle Metabolism in Exercise and Diabetes. Advances in Experimental Medicine and Biology Volume 441, 1998, pp 1-16

2 Insulin Biosynthesis, Secretion, Structure and Structure-Activity Relationship Michael Weiss, Donald F. Steiner, Louis H. Philipson,and Insulin signaling and action: glucose, lipids, protein Cai Li, Bei B. Zhang, In ENDOTEXT downloaded from www.endotext.org,. Leslie J De Groot, Kathleen Dungan (eds) 2015

3 Jumpertz JC, Thearle MS , Bunt JC Exercise Regulation Of Glucose Transport In Skeletal Muscle.Metabolism. 2010; 59 (10):1396-1401. doi10-1016/J Metabol.2010.01.006 \

4 Sleep loss: a novel risk factor for insulin resistance and Type 2 diabetes, Spiegel K, Knutson K, Leproult R, et al. J Appl Physiol 2005; 99(5): 2008-19:DOI10.1152/japplphysiol.00660.2005

5 What is Normal Glucose? – Continuous Glucose Monitoring Data from Healthy Subjects, Christiansen, Prof. J. S., presented at the EASD Annual Meeting, Copenhagen 09-06-2013

6 King P, Peacock,1, Donnelly P The UK Prospective Diabetes Study (UKPDS): clinical and therapeutic implications for type 2 diabetes. Br J Clin Pharmacol.1999 Nov; 48(5): 643–648.doi: 10.1046/j.1365-2125.1999.00092.xPMCID: PMC201435

7 Implications of the Diabetes Control and Complications Trial, Diabetes Care January 2002 25:suppl 1 s25-s27;doi:10.2337/diabetes care..2007; S25: 1935-5548

8 David M. Nathan, DCCT/EDIC 30th Anniversary Summary Findings: The Diabetes Control and Complications Trial/Epidemiology of Diabetes Interventions and Complications Study at 30 Years: Overview, Diabetes Care 2014; 37(1): 9-16; doi:10.2337/dc13-2112 1935-5548

9 Gregg EW, Li Y, Wang J et al. Changes in Diabetes–Related Complications in the United States, 1990-2010, N Eng J Med 2014; 370 (16):1514-1523.

10 The Diabetes Control and Complications Trial/ Epidemiology of Diabetes Interventions and Complications (DCCT/EDIC) Study Research Group. Intensive Diabetes Treatment and Cardiovascular Disease in Patients with Type 1 Diabetes. N Engl J Med 2005;353(12):2643-53: DOI: 10.1056/NEJMoa052187.

11 DCCT Study Group, N Engl J Med 1993; 329:977-86. Reichard P, N Engl J Med 1993; 329:304-9. Primary Outcome. Development or Progression. Retinopathy. Nephropathy

12 Holman RR, Paul SK, Bethel MA, et al.10-Year Follow-up of Intensive Glucose Control in Type 2 Diabetes N Engl J Med 2008; 359:1577-1589October 9, 2008DOI:10.1056/NEJMoa0806470

13 Orchard TJ, Temprosa M, Goldberg R, et al. The Effect of Metformin and Intensive Lifestyle Intervention on the Metabolic Syndrome: The Diabetes Prevention Program Randomized Trial FREE. Ann Intern Med. 2005;142(8):611-619. doi:10.7326/0003-4819-142-8-200504190-00009

14 www.diabetesdaily.com/blog/2012/04/the-meter-took-power-from-the-doctor-gave-it-to-the- patient

15 From the National Glycohemoglobin Standardization Program, downloaded from www.ngsp. org/bground.asp 6-30-2014

16 Colberg SR, Hernandez MJ, Shahzad F. Blood glucose responses to type, intensity, duration, and timing of exercise. Diabetes Care.2013; 36(10):e177.J

17 Taylor LA1, Rachman SJ. Behav Med. 1988 Jun;11(3):279-91.The effects of blood sugar level changes on cognitive function, affective state, and s;omatic symptoms.

18 American Diabetes Association. Diabetes Care. 2015 38:S41-S48; doi:10.2337/dc15-S010

19 AACE/ACE Comprehensive Diabetes Management Algorithm 2015 Endocr Pract. 2015; 21:438-447.

20 Koivisto V, Felig P. Effects of Leg Exercise on Insulin Absorption in Diabetic Patients N Engl J Med 1978; 298:79-83 DOI: 10.1056/NEJM197801122980205

21 To Err Is Human Building a Safer Health System, : Institute of Medicine: 2000

22 Russell SJ, El-Khatib FH, Sinha M., et al. Outpatient Glycemic Control with a Bionic Pancreas in Type 1 Diabetes. N Engl J Med 2014; 371:313-325

23 Ferrannini E.The Target of Metformin in Type 2 Diabetes N Engl J Med. 2014;371(16):1547-8.

24 "U.S. Food and Drug Administration." Rosiglitazone-containing Diabetes Medicines: Drug Safety Communication. FDA, 25 Nov. 2013. Web. 16 Feb. 2015.

25 Garber AJ. Long-Acting Glucagon-Like Peptide 1 Receptor Agonists: A Review Of Their Efficacy And Tolerability. Diabetes Care. 2011;34 Suppl 2:S279-84.

26 Polonski, W.H., Fisher, L., Earles, J, et al Assessing psychological stress in diabetes. Diabete Care. 2005; 28: 626 – 631

27 Admiraal WM, Celik F, Gerdes VE et al., Ethnic Differences in Weight Loss and Diabetes Remission After Bariatric Surgery: A meta-analysis Diabetes Care. 2012; 35(9): 1951–1958. 10.2337/dc12-0260.PMCID: PMC3424999

28 The Action to Control Cardiovascular Risk in Diabetes Study Group. Effects of Intensive Glucose Lowering in Type 2 Diabetes.N Engl J Med 2008; 358:2545-2559June 12, 2008DOI: 10.1056/NEJMoa0802743

29 Cryer P. Banting lecture: hypoglycemia, limiting factor in the management of IDDM. Diabetes.1994;43: 1378–1389.

30 Kahneman D. Thinking, Fast and Slow. Farrar, Strauss and Giroux , New York, 2013

31 Whorle HJ, Neuman Z, Impact of fasting and postprandial Effect of Moderate-Intensity Exercise Versus Activities of Daily Living on 24-Hour Blood Glucose Homeostasis in Male Patients With Type 2 Diabetes. Diabetes Care.2013;36(11):3448-3453.doi:10.2337/dc12-2620

32 Joslin, E. Diabetic Manual for the Mutual Use Of Doctor And Patient, 6TH ed. Lea & Febiger, Philadelphia.1937 pg. 14.

33 Loomis AL. Textbook of Practical Medicine, 2nd ed. William Wood & Company, New York 1984 pg. 878.

34 Nainggolan, Lisa. Life Expectancy Greatly Improved in Type 1 Diabetes. (2013). Retrieved from www.medscape.com/viewarticle/811610 on 9/23/2014.

35 Early Treatment Diabetic Retinopathy Study Research Group Photocoagulation for diabetic macular edema. Early Treatment Diabetic Retinopathy Study report number 1. Arch Ophthalmol 1985. 1031796–1806.1806 [PubMed]

36 Loon RL. Diabetic Kidney Disease: Preventing Dialysis and Transplantation Clinical Diabetes 2003;21(2):55-62. doi: 10.2337/ diaclin.21.2.55

37 www.nchealthliteracy.org/toolkit/tool5.pdf

38 Charles Duhigg, The Power of Habit: Why We Do What We Do in Life and Business. Random House, New York

39 Baumeister RF. Bratslavsky E, Muraven M.et al. Ego depletion: Is the Active Self: a limited resource? J Personality Social Psychology, 1998;74(5), 1252-1265

40 Job V. Walton GM, Bernecker K, et al. Beliefs About Willpower Determine The Impact Of Glucose On Self-Control, PNAS 2013; 110 (37): 14837-14842-ahead of print August 19, 2013,doi:10.1073/pnas.1313475110

41 Wansink, Brian and Matthew M. Cheney (2005), "Super Bowls: Serving Bowl Size and Food Consumption," JAMA, 293:14, 1727–1728.

42 Van Cauter E, Polonsky KS, Scheen AJ. Roles of circadian rhythmicity and sleep in human glucose regulation. Endocr Rev. 1997;18:716–738

43 Tools to Face the Psychological Demands of Diabetes.The Behavioral Diabetes Institute [Internet]. Available from: behavioraldiabetesin-stitute.org.

44 Nash J. Diabetes and Wellbeing. Wiley-Blackwell. 2013. Hoboken

45 Medici F et al. Concordance rate for type II diabetes mellitus in monozygotic twins: actuarial analysis. Diabetologia 1999;42: 146-50.

46 Greenberger, Dennis and Padesky, Christine Mind Over Mood. Guilford Press Greenberger, Dennis and Padesky, Christine Mind Over Mood. Guilford Press, 1995. New York

47 Tversky A, and Kahneman D . Taken from Judgment Under Certainty: Heuristics and Biases. 1974, 185., Thinking, Fast and Slow by Daniel Kahneman

48 Laird JD. Self-attribution of emotion: the effects of expressive behavior on the quality of emotional experience. J Pers Soc Psychol. 1974 Apr;29(4):475-86.

49 Ma SH, Teasdale JD. Mindfulness-based cognitive therapy for depression: replication and explora-tion of differential relapse prevention effects. J Consult Clin Psychol. 2004; 72(1):31-40.

50 Farb NA, Segal ZV, Mayberg H, et al. Attending to the present: mindfulness meditation reveals distinct neural modes of self-reference. Soc Cogn Affect Neurosci. 2007;2(4):313-22

51 www.behavioraldiabetesinstitute.org

52 Pentland A. Social Physics, Penguin Press, New York, 2014

53 Pugh KH. Sharing Hidden Know-How Josey-Bass, 2011 San Francisco Pg 19-30

54 Heisler M Overview of Peer Support Models to Improve Diabetes Self-Management and Clinical Outcomes Diabetes Spectrum 2007; 20(4):214-221. Doi : 10.2337/diaspect.20.4.214

Index

A

A1c levels
basal insulin and, 79
definition of, 39
depression and, 171, 172
DPP-4 inhibitors and, 61
flaws of, 126, 128
goals for, 118
grief and, 107
Health Effectiveness Data and
Information Sets (HEDIS)
and, 139
heart disease and, 83
in-range monitoring
compared to, 126–128
medications and, 51, 78, 79
post-meal blood sugar and, 128
stress and, 72, 73, 118
targets, 39–40, 128
ACCORD (Action to Control
Cardiovascular Risk in
Diabetes), 83
adaptations
children and, 119
in-range monitoring 126–128
intuition and, 125
safety and, 121–123
slowing digestion, 129–130
alcohol, 88
Allen, Frederick, 50
allergies, to insulin, 52
alpha-glucosidase inhibitors, 61
amputations, 19, 21, 72
analog insulin, 130–131
antidepressants, 81, 173
anxiety, 24–25
Apidra insulin, 54, 131
artificial pancreas, 58

B

basal-bolus insulin therapy, 52
basal insulin, 52, 53, 57, 78–79
Baumeister, Roy, 145
Behavioral Diabetes Institute, 167
Big Blue Test, 46
Blood Glucose Awareness
Training (BGAT), 85

blood glucose meters. *See also*
continuous glucose meters;
monitoring; testing.
accuracy of, 104
health care industry and, 35,
110
introduction to, 37–38
testing locations, 38
test strips for, 38, 104
usage instructions, 38
blood pressure, 140
blood sugar. *See* high blood
sugar; low blood sugar.
bolus insulin, 52, 53, 79–80
Borushek, Allan, 74
brain, 47, 84, 123
breastfeeding, 109
Brosh, Allie, 171
burnout, 169–170

C

CalorieKing (Allan Borushek),
74
carbohydrates
alpha-glucosidase inhibitors
and, 61
counting, 43–44, 74–75
digestion of, 43, 61, 74, 89,
129, 130
fats and, 44
fiber and, 43
high blood sugar and, 43, 52,
73, 74–75, 113, 114, 130
insulin and, 54, 62, 75, 78, 88,
94–95
low blood sugar and, 91, 92,
94–95
weight loss and, 63
cardiac stress tests, 46
cellular function, 66–67
Certified Diabetes Educators
(CDE), 17, 143
Children with Diabetes website,
182
Cognitive Behavioral Therapy
(CBT), 154–155

complications
amputations, 19, 21, 72
awareness of, 19–21
fat processing, 21
genetics and, 17
macrovascular, 20
micro-changes, 20
microvascular, 20
pain, 20–21
tingling, 20–21
confounders
accounting for, 110
addressing, 118
blood glucose meters as, 104
breastfeeding, 109
Dawn Phenomenon and, 113
device failure as, 104
emotions, 106
fixing, 109–110
grief, 107
identifying, 70–71
low blood sugar and, 104
medications, 71, 103
menstrual cycle, 105
pain as, 71, 104, 105–106
removing, 109
rhythm disruptions, 108
sleep, 104
stress, 71, 72–73, 104
unseen triggers, 107, 113
continuous glucose meters
(CGMs). *See also* blood glucose
meters.
accuracy of, 39
device failure, 104
hypoglycemia unawareness
and, 94, 95
in-range monitoring with, 99,
126, 128
insurance coverage for, 184
usage, 39
sensors, 10, 39
C-Peptide tests, 22, 42, 81, 82

D

Dawn Phenomenon, 33,
113–114

DCCT (Diabetes Control and
Complications Trial), 83
Dealing with Diabetes Burnout
(Ginger Vieira), 169
depression
A1c levels and, 171, 172
antidepressants, 173
balanced approach to,
172–173
exercise and, 173
hormonal triggers, 171
dextrose, 92
Diabetes and Wellbeing (Jen
Nash), 155
Diabetes Burnout (Bill Polonsky),
169
Diabetes Control and Complication Trial (DCCT), 18
Diabetes Daily website, 7, 182
Diabetes Hands Foundation, 81
Diabetes Prevention Program, 19
diabetic ketoacidosis (DKA), 18,
22, 100
diagnoses
type 1 diabetes, 22, 81, 82
type 2 diabetes, 21
diet. *See* foods; weight loss.
dietitians, 142
distress
burnout and, 169–170
signs of, 167–168
survey for, 167
therapists and, 168–169
doctors. *See also* health care
team.
burnout and, 170
checklist, 137–140
emotional issues and, 162
endocrinologists, 95
food diaries and, 45
health care industry and, 36
medication and, 77, 78, 81,
103, 138, 181
"noncompliance" and, 23
performance incentives for,
183–184
roles of, 141–142
self-care compared to, 135–136

support network and, 174–176
"teach back" method,
140–141, 175
DPP-4 inhibitors, 61
Duhigg, Charles, 144

E

eAG ("estimated average
glucose"), 40
EDIC study, 18
emotions
Cognitive Behavioral Therapy
(CBT), 154–155
as confounder, 106
coping strategies, 161–162
depression, 170–173
diabetes management and, 17
"flourishing" mindset, 158–160
food and, 156
guilt, 157–158
mental health issues, 162–163
mindfulness, 163–164
negative coping strategies,
161–162
reframing thoughts, 154–157
ruts, 153
self-control, 164–165
self-forgiveness, 158
shame, 157–158
sharing, 160
uncertainty, 152–154
empowerment, 23–24
EsTuDiabetes website, 182
exercise
Big Blue Test, 46
depression and, 173
emergencies and, 123
habits for, 147–148, 151
heart disease and, 132
high blood sugar and, 46,
75–76, 77
importance of, 45
insulin and, 45, 76, 132
intense, 46
light to moderate, 46
low blood sugar and, 87
safety and, 132
weight loss and, 132
eye exams, 139

F

Facebook, 182
fast-acting insulin. *See*
rapid-acting insulin.
fat cells, 48
fats, 44, 91–92
fiber, 43
Fogg, B.J., 150
foods
absorption, 88
carbohydrates, 50
diaries, 45
dietitians, 142
emotions and, 156
fats, 44
fiber, 43
Glycemic Index (GI), 129–130
healthy habits for, 148–150
individual reactions to, 67,
68–69
multipliers and, 101–102
nighttime and, 113
pizza, 44, 119–120
post-meal blood sugar, 128
protein, 20, 44, 47, 91–92
restaurant strategies, 148–149
Rule of Threes, 69, 74
slowing digestion of, 129–130
Frankl, Viktor, 133

G

GAD antibodies tests, 22
genetics, 157
gestational diabetes, 22
GLP-1s, 60
glucagon injections, 92–93
glucose meters. *See* blood
glucose meters.
Glycemic Index (GI), 129–130
glycogen, 44
glynides, 61
Greater Good Science Center, 163
Greenberg, Riva, 158–160
grief, 107

H

habits
environmental changes and,
146–148
foods and, 148–150
friends and, 150–151

peer mentor groups and, 182
reward and, 144
self-control and, 145–146
sleep and, 149
unfamiliarity and, 149–150
weight loss and, 148–149
Hall, Gary, 46
health care industry
appeals to, 184
blood glucose meters and, 35,
110
dependence on, 9
disconnect with, 23
doctors and, 36
health care workers and, 143
Health Effectiveness Data and
Information Sets (HEDIS),
138–139
prevention and, 36
reform of, 183–184
as "sick care," 23–24, 36, 183
health care team. *See also*
doctors.
Certified Diabetes Educators
(CDE), 143
checklists for, 136–140
dietitians, 142
family, 143
friends, 143
health care workers, 143
medical histories, 138
medications and, 138
nurse practitioners, 142
nurses, 142
peers, 143
physician's assistants, 142
Health Effectiveness Data and
Information Sets (HEDIS),
138–139
heart disease
emotional suppression and, 160
high blood sugar and, 46, 77,
132
metformin and, 59
post-meal blood sugar and, 128
risks of, 139
TZDs and, 60
Hemoglobin A1c. *See* A1c levels.
Hernandez, Manny, 81
high blood sugar
basal insulin, 78–79
bolus insulin, 79–80

carbohydrates and, 43, 52, 73,
74–75, 113, 114, 130
cellular activity and, 66–67
complications of, 15–16
Dawn Phenomenon and, 33
diabetic ketoacidosis (DKA)
and, 18
dietary changes and, 73
digestion and, 74
exercise and, 46, 75–76, 77
heart disease and, 46, 77, 132
low blood sugar and, 27–28
medications for, 76–78, 78–80
misdiagnosis and, 81–82
monitoring, 69–70
multiple medications for, 80
nighttime and, 112–113
non-insulin treatments for,
77–78
pain and, 105–106
Rule of Threes and 67–69, 73
stress and, 29–30, 70, 71, 72–73
hormones
depression and, 171
digestion and, 47
GLP-1 hormones, 61
low blood sugar and, 27, 89
rhythms, 54, 102, 105
sleep and, 54
stress and, 62
Hughes, Elizabeth Evans, 50
Humalog, 131
Humulin, 55
Humulin N, 55
Humulin R, 130
hydration, 41–42
hypoglycemia. *See* low blood
sugar.

I

inhaled insulin, 56
in-range monitoring, 99, 126–128
Institute of Medicine, 54
insulin. *See also* medication.
A1c levels and, 51
allergies to, 52
analog insulin, 130–131
Apidra, 54, 131
bad insulin, 103
basal-bolus therapy, 52
basal insulin, 52, 53, 57, 78–79
bolus insulin, 52, 53, 79–80

carbohydrates and, 54, 62, 75, 78, 88, 94–95
digestion and, 74
discovery of, 50, 134
dosage strategies, 119–120
exercise and, 45, 76, 132
history of, 50
Humalog, 54, 131
Humulin, 55
Humulin N, 55
Humulin R, 130
inhaled insulin, 56
injection tips, 52–53
insulin pens, 56
insulin pumps, 52, 56–57, 104, 181
intermediate-acting insulin (NPH), 56
long-acting insulin, 54
low blood sugar and, 94
mixed insulin, 55–56
multiple medications and, 81
muscle injections, 52–53, 88
natural production of, 51
Novolin, 55
Novolin R, 130
Novolog, 54, 131
NPH, 55, 79, 131
quality of, 13
rapid-acting, 54–55, 78–79, 131
Rule of Threes and, 79
safety, 49, 94–95, 131
short-acting, 55
side effects of, 134
speeding up, 130–131
stacking, 80
type 1 diabetes and, 49, 55, 78, 79
type 2 diabetes and, 55
weight loss and, 63
Insulin Pumps and Continuous Glucose Monitoring (Francine R. Kaufman), 57
insurance. *See* health care industry.
intermediate-acting insulin (NPH), 56
interstitial fluid, 39
intestines, 47, 60, 61

J
Johnson, Nicole, 159
Joslin, Elliott, 65, 134–135

K
Kahneman, Daniel, 123, 164
Kaufman, Francine R., 57
ketones, 41–42, 62
kidneys, 20, 48, 139
Kirk-Macri, Ellen, 23

L
lab-drawn blood sugar tests, 38–39
lactic acidosis, 59
LADA ("latent autoimmune diabetes of adulthood"), 23
Lancet, The journal, 50
LDL cholesterol, 139
"legacy of health," 17–18
Lincoln, Abraham, 12
liver
    alcohol and, 88
    basal insulin and, 52
    bolus insulin and, 52
    fat storage, 48
    GLP-1 and, 60
    gluconeogenesis, 47
    hormone rhythms and, 54, 89
    metformin and, 59
    stress and, 47
    sugar production, 47
    sulfonylureas and, 60
    TZDs and, 60
low blood sugar
    alcohol and, 88
    awareness of, 85, 93–94
    Blood Glucose Awareness Training (BGAT), 85
    carbohydrates and, 91, 92, 94–95
    complications of, 16–17
    continuous glucose meters and, 94, 97
    damage from, 87
    dementia similarities to, 86–87
    dextrose and, 92
    digestion and, 89
    exercise and, 87
    food absorption and, 88

glucagon injections and, 92–93
high blood sugar and, 27–28
hormonal irregularities and, 27, 89
hypoglycemia unawareness, 84, 85
morning and, 112
nighttime, 112–113
preparation for, 91
quick treatment of, 91–92
reactions to, 84, 85
recordkeeping and, 34
studies of, 83
symptoms and, 115
unconsciousness and, 85, 92–93

M
macrovascular complications, 20
medication. *See also* insulin.
    A1c levels and, 51, 78, 79
    alpha-glucosidase inhibitors, 61
    antidepressants, 81
    as confounders, 103
    doctors and, 77, 78, 81, 103, 138, 181
    DPP-4 inhibitors, 61
    GLP-1s, 60
    glucagon injections, 92–93
    glynides, 61
    health care teams and, 138
    intermediate-acting insulin (NPH), 56
    lactic acidosis and, 59
    low blood sugar and, 94
    metformin, 49, 59, 78
    multiple medications, 80–81
    peer mentor groups and, 181
    quality of, 13
    questions to ask, 48–49
    risks of, 59
    Rule of Threes, 78
    SGLT-2s, 61
    slowing digestion with, 130
    steroids, 81
    sulfonylureas, 59–60, 132
    TZDs, 60
Medtronic company, 58
menstrual cycle, 105
metformin, 49, 59, 78

microvascular complications, 20
mixed insulins, 55–56
monitoring. *See also* blood glucose meters; testing.
    A1c levels, 39–40
    afternoon lows, 115
    bedtime, 116
    blood glucose meters, 37–38, 100, 110
    consistency of results, 112
    continuous glucose meters (CGMs), 13, 39, 126, 128
    Dawn Phenomenon and, 33, 113–114
    eAG ("estimated average glucose"), 40
    frequency of, 69–70, 110, 111–112
    importance of, 110
    in-range monitoring, 99, 126–128
    lab-drawn blood sugar tests, 38–39
    lunch to evening, 114
    nighttime, 112–113
    timing of, 111–112
    urine and, 99
multipliers, 101–102

N
Nash, Jen, 155
National Committee for Quality Assurance (NCQA), 138
nerve damage, 20–21
Novolin, 55
Novolin R, 130
Novolog, 54, 131
NPH (neutral protamine Hagedorn) insulin, 55, 79, 131
nurse practitioners, 142
nurses, 142

P
pain
    awareness of, 20–21
    basal insulin and, 81
    as confounder, 71, 104, 105–106
    injections and, 52, 56, 88
    lack of, 20–21, 46
    stress and, 104

peer mentor groups, 179–182

physician's assistants, 142

pizza, 44, 119–120

Polonsky, William, 167, 169

Power of Habit, The (Charles Duhigg), 144

pre-diabetes, 22

prescribing information (PI), 54

proteins, 44, 91–92

Pugh, Kate, 181–182

Pumping Insulin (John Walsh and Ruth Roberts), 57

R

rapid-acting insulin, 54–55, 79–80, 131

recordkeeping, 34, 35, 45

retinal eye exams, 139

reversal, 19

Roberts, Ruth, 57

Roizen, Dr., 150

Rule of Threes
foods, 69, 74
high blood sugar and, 67–69, 73
insulin dosage and, 79
introduction to, 67–68
medications and, 78
rapidly changing patterns and, 70

S

safety
decision-making and, 27, 121, 122
exercise, 132
insulin and, 49, 94–95, 131
treatment decisions and, 27

self-control, 145–146

SGLT-2s, 61

short-acting insulin, 55

sleep, 104, 112, 149

steroids, 81

stress
A1c levels and, 72, 73, 118
as confounder, 29–30, 104
high blood sugar and, 29–30, 70, 71, 72–73
management of, 62

sulfonylureas, 59–60, 132

support network
accountability, 182
boundaries for, 177
colleagues, 176–177, 178–179
communication with, 178–179, 181–182
doctor, 174–176
family, 176–177
friends, 176–177
habits and, 182
negative comments, 176–177, 178
online sources, 182
peer mentor groups, 179–182
political representatives and, 184
putting yourself first, 183–184

T

"teach back" method, 140–141, 175

testing. *See also* blood glucose meters; monitoring.
blood pressure, 140
cardiac stress, 46
C-Peptide, 22, 42, 81, 82
GAD antibodies, 22
ketones, 41
kidney health, 139
LDL cholesterol, 139

Thinking, Fast and Slow (Daniel Kahneman), 123, 164

Thriving with Diabetes website, 57, 167, 169, 171, 182, 184

"time in range." *See* in-range monitoring.

TuDiabetes website, 182

type 1 diabetes
age and, 22, 81
basal insulin for, 78
C-Peptide test, 22, 42
Diabetes Control and Complication Trial (DCCT), 18
diabetic ketoacidosis, 18
diagnosing, 22, 81, 82
GAD antibodies test, 22
risk of complications, 17, 18
in-range monitoring of, 99–100
insulin for, 49, 55, 78, 79

insulin production and, 15, 42, 51, 81
insulin pumps for, 57, 159
introduction to, 22
ketones and, 41
LADA as, 23
Lancet article, 50
medications for, 77
misdiagnosing, 81, 82
mixed insulin and, 56
rapid-acting insulin for, 55, 79
sleep and, 113

type 2 diabetes
basal insulin for, 79
diabetic ketoacidosis, 18
diagnosing, 21
fats and, 44
genetics and, 157
gestational diabetes and, 22
guilt and, 157
insulin for, 55
insulin production and, 42, 51
introduction to, 21–22
ketones and, 41, 42
medications for, 49, 51, 77
metformin, 49
misdiagnosing, 81
mixed insulin for, 55
non-insulin treatments for, 77–78
pre-diabetes and, 22
prevalence of, 21
rapid-acting insulin for, 55, 79
reversal of, 19
risk of complications, 17
sleep and, 113
shame and, 157
United Kingdom Prospective Diabetes Study (UKPDS), 18
weight loss surgery and, 63

TZDs, 60

U

United Kingdom Prospective Diabetes Study (UKPDS), 18

V

Vieira, Ginger, 169

W

Walsh, John, 57

websites
CalorieKing, 74
Children with Diabetes, 182
Diabetes Daily, 7, 182
EsTuDiabetes, 182
Facebook, 182
Thriving with Diabetes, 57, 167, 169, 171, 182, 184
TuDiabetes, 182

weight loss
calorie restrictions, 62
carbohydrates and, 63
exercise and, 132
"flourishing" mindset and, 159–160
insulin and, 63, 132
portions size and, 148, 149
restaurants and, 148–149
surgery for, 63–64
water loss, 132

Y

Youngstown Pump Club, 179–180, 181

Z

Zabell, Elizabeth, 7